T0231313

James W. Cooper
Editor

Geriatric Drug Therapy Interventions

Geriatric Drug Therapy Interventions has been co-published simultaneously as *Journal of Geriatric Drug Therapy*, Volume 11, Number 4 1997.

Pre-publication REVIEWS, COMMENTARIES, EVALUATIONS . . .

Geriatric Drug Therapy Interventions

Geriatric Drug Therapy Interventions has been co-published simultaneously as *Journal of Geriatric Drug Therapy,* Volume 11, Number 4 1997.

The *Journal of Geriatric Drug Therapy* Monographs/"Separates"

Geriopharmacotherapy in Home Health Care: New Frontiers in Pharmaceutical Care, edited by Steven R. Moore

Antiinfectives in the Elderly, edited by James W. Cooper

Antivirals in the Elderly, edited by James W. Cooper

Geriatric Drug Therapy Interventions, edited by James W. Cooper

These books were published simultaneously as special thematic issues of the *Journal of Geriatric Drug Therapy* and are available bound separately. Visit Haworth's website at http://www.haworth.com to search our on-line catalog for complete tables of contents and ordering information for these and other publications. Or call 1-800-HAWORTH (outside US/Canada: 607-722-5857), Fax: 1-800-895-0582 (outside US/Canada: 607-771-0012), or e-mail getinfo@haworth.com

Geriatric Drug Therapy Interventions

James W. Cooper
Editor

Geriatric Drug Therapy Interventions has been co-published simultaneously as *Journal of Geriatric Drug Therapy,* Volume 11, Number 4 1997.

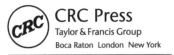

CRC Press
Taylor & Francis Group
Boca Raton London New York

CRC Press is an imprint of the
Taylor & Francis Group, an **informa** business

Geriatric Drug Therapy Interventions

CONTENTS

ABOUT THE EDITOR

James W. Cooper, PharmPhD, is Professor of Pharmacy Practice at the University of Georgia College of Pharmacy in Athens, Georgia, and Assistant Clinical Professor of Family Medicine at the Medical College of Georgia. He is the author or editor of 30 books and monographs, ten book chapters, and over 400 research and professional publications. He teaches, practices, and conducts research in consultant pharmacy with geriatric patients in ambulatory and long-term care settings. The Editor of the *Journal of Geriatric Drug Therapy,* Dr. Cooper is a board-certified pharmacotherapy specialist and a Fellow of the American Societies of Consultant Pharmacists and Health Systems Pharmacists. In 1981, he was a special advisor to the White House Conference on Aging. He is the recipient of numerous national awards for his work, and has received more than a million dollars in funding to support his research and service.

Introduction

This text is devoted to geriatric drug therapy interventions. The editor reviews interventions and issues with medication usage in the older patient. Fincham and Hunter present data on community pharmacist interventions with geriatric patients over a one month period in 25 pharmacies. If the standard of care that was utilized and savings of almost $1300 per intervention with geriatric patients were extrapolated to a national sample of geriatric patients over a year there would be no need for budget cuts in medicaid and medicare that are currently being explored in Washington.

Chisholm, Taylor and Hawkins studied interventions in geriatric patients by Pharm. D. students on clerkships and found a positive impact on patient care in a tertiary care center. The editor investigated the interventions by one consultant pharmacist over a one-year period in one nursing facility. He found that more cost savings were lost by refusal to accept a small proportion (9%) of intervention recommendations than was gained by acceptance of 91% of those recommendations. If the $241 per patient per year saving is projected to the estimated 1.7 million nursing facility residents in the US the savings could be some $410 million dollars. The Fleetwood project that is currently being conducted by the American Society of Consultant Pharmacists will further determine possible costs savings to the health care system by these interventions.

The editor concludes with a case report of the costs of intervention failure in a single patient that resulted in over $50,000 in excess costs to the health care system.

James W. Cooper

[Haworth indexing entry note]: "Introduction." Cooper, James W. Published in *Geriatric Drug Therapy Interventions* (ed: James W. Cooper) The Pharmaceutical Products Press, an imprint of The Haworth Press, Inc., 1997, p. 1. Single or multiple copies of this article are available for a fee from The Haworth Document Delivery Service [1-800-342-9678, 9:00 a.m. - 5:00 p.m. (EST). E-mail address: getinfo@haworth.com].

REVIEW ARTICLE

Geriatric Drug Therapy Interventions

James W. Cooper

SUMMARY. Geriatric drug therapy interventions involve the encouragement of appropriate therapy and prevention of problems with medications. Exponentially rising health care costs of the elderly have brought radical suggestions for rationing of health care. The place of drug therapy in holistic care of the older patient should be in the context of an increased awareness of the self-care concepts of "wellness." Drug-related problems of non-compliance and adverse drug reaction and interactions may influence the need for admission of up to one-third of hospitalizations and one-half of nursing home placements of older adults. Additionally, drug-related problems occur across all levels of progressive patient care. In the nursing facility, two-thirds of patients have been shown to have a drug-related

James W. Cooper, PhD, BCPS, FASCP, FASHP, is Professor of Pharmacy Practice, College of Pharmacy, and Gerontology Faculty, University of Georgia, Athens, GA 30602, and Assistant Clinical Professor, Department of Family Medicine, Medical College of Georgia, Augusta, GA 30912.

This article was presented in part at the Third International Congress on Geriatric Pharmacotherapy and Nutrition, Alicante, Spain, 1994.

[Haworth co-indexing entry note]: "Geriatric Drug Therapy Interventions." Cooper, James W. Co-published simultaneously in *Journal of Geriatric Drug Therapy* (The Pharmaceutical Products Press, an imprint of The Haworth Press, Inc.) Vol. 11, No. 4, 1997, pp. 3-26; and: *Geriatric Drug Therapy Interventions* (ed: James W. Cooper) The Pharmaceutical Products Press, an imprint of The Haworth Press, Inc., 1997, pp. 3-26. Single or multiple copies of this article are available for a fee from The Haworth Document Delivery Service [1-800-342-9678, 9:00 a.m. - 5:00 p.m. (EST). E-mail address: getinfo@haworth.com].

3

problem up to every other month during their length of stay. Under-recognition of patient problems as well as misdiagnosis studies have pointed out areas where drug therapy outcomes could be improved, especially in the areas of malnutrition, depression, osteoporosis and dementia. The Food and Drug Administration has proposed new guidelines for all drugs to include a pharmacokinetic screen to assure that geriatric patients can have safe levels of newer agents. Insidious adverse drug effects of increased falls and fractures as well as pressure ulcers due to psychoactive drugs, NSAID-associated gastritis and gastrointestinal bleeding, drug-induced delirium and incontinence and constipation are being detected. Managed care may offer less than optimal care when compared with fee-for-service plans for health care of the elderly. Interventions in geriatric drug therapy can improve drug adherence and reduce adverse drug reactions as well as contribute to improved disease state management in the geriatric patient. *[Article copies available for a fee from The Haworth Document Delivery Service: 1-800-342-9678. E-mail address: getinfo@haworth.com]*

KEYWORDS: geriatric, drug therapy, drug-related problems, interventions

I. HEALTH CARE COSTS OF THE ELDERLY

Drug therapy is the most frequently used therapeutic intervention in geriatric patients. Unfortunately, a recent report from the U.S. House of Representatives Select Committee on Aging entitled "Emptying the Elderly's Pocketbook–Growing Impact of Rising Health Care Costs," produced disturbing results: American elderly out-of-pocket expenses for health and long-term care will reach 20% or more of their mean income in the 1990's, up from 12% of disposable income in 1977. The report argued that a comprehensive system of cost-containment must be employed if health care costs are to be kept affordable for all Americans.[1]

It should be noted that fully 95% of American elderly over 65 years of age are ambulatory and capable of some form of self-care; 5% are institutionalized in nursing homes and acute care hospitals. In a further study on "the aging of America: impact on health care costs," the rapid growth of the oldest old age groups (greater than 85 years of age) will have a major impact on future health care costs for Medicare, nursing homes, dementia and hip fractures. Projecting forward to the year 2040, Medicare will increase six-fold; the cost of dementia treatment alone will exceed the 1985 American budget deficit (150 billion dollars).[2]

The highest priority health and drug therapy needs of the elderly are noted in Table 1.[3] The advent of managed care does not bode well for the overall health outcomes of the elderly. A recent 4-year study found that the elderly and poor chronically ill had worse physical health outcomes under a health maintenance organization (HMO) than in a fee-for-service plan.[4] On consideration of the ways in which patients can be treated, or modalities of therapy in holistic or "total" care, there are what are referred to as "wellness" and "treatment" modalities: wellness modalities include "tender loving care" (TLC), nutrition, and physical exercise or activity. The public esteem of any health professional is in direct proportion to the degree that we project a "caring attitude" as well as help to ameliorate disease conditions. Proper nutrition is essential to wellness, as is adequate physical activity.

Treatment modalities include medications, surgery, radiation, and counseling. The counseling modality is of course also an integral part of care and attention (TLC).

One concept of why people become "less than well" is that many believe that a large percentage of problems seen by primary care providers are due to: abuse of alcohol and other legitimate and illegal chemicals; abuse of tobacco products; improper diet quantity and quality; lack of belief in self or absence of TLC support system and lack of belief in something greater than self, as well as lack of appropriate physical activity.

II. DRUG-RELATED PROBLEMS (DRPs) OF MISUSE AND ADVERSE REACTION

In terms of drug-related problems of the elderly, it has been found that up to one-third of the elderly, compared to one-fifth of all age groups have drug-related problems that influence their need for hospital admissions.[5] Drug-related problems (DRPs) may be defined as any unwanted consequence of the drug utilization process.

TABLE 1. Highest Priority Health and Drug Therapy Needs of the Elderly[3]

Preventive Care

1. Recognition that age-related changes may not require drugs.
2. Basic information about prescription and OTC drugs, their benefits and risks, alternatives to drug use, and medical and other health care services.
3. Understanding the values and myths of home remedies and development of a cautious attitude towards fads in health care.
4. Acceptance of drug therapy as a potentially necessary and beneficial part of aging and encouragement of compliance with necessary drug therapy.
5. Maintenance of dignity and respect in the health care system.
6. Maintenance of a complete drug history and drug regimen review process.
7. Communications with service providers that are clear and adapted to receptive or expressive needs of the elderly.
8. Referral to medical or other health care services.

Chronic Care

1. Recognition that age-related changes may not require drugs.
2. Information on alternatives or supplements to drug use, values and myths of home remedies, and drug-diet interactions.
3. Provision of and appropriate storage of medicines.
4. Maintenance of a complete drug history.
5. Insistence on review and monitoring of the drug treatment plan.
6. Information about drugs being taken, the do's and don'ts of drug therapy, cooperation with the drug treatment plan, when to contact service providers and what to report.
7. Assessing patient comprehension and pharmacist understanding of therapeutic objectives and rationality of the treatment plan.
8. Identification of noncompliance and adverse effects of medications.
9. Ability to appropriately use appliances and devices.

Acute Care

1. Careful evaluation of patient problems, rationality of drug prescribing, and recommendation/provision of drug and non-drug therapies.
2. Maintenance of a complete drug history, and monitoring and review of the treatment plan.
3. Identification of adverse medication effects.
4. Appreciation of the value of medication and its effect.

Although many events can and do occur in this process, from the assessment of a patient's problems to the therapeutic outcome in that patient, the two main DRP classifications are drug misuse and adverse drug reaction or interaction. When both types of problems are simultaneously assessed in the same patient population entering a hospital, the frequency of those problems has been demonstrated to increase with age.[5]

Admissions to Hospitals and In-Hospital DRPs

When a complete drug history of drug use prior to admission is done on all patients entering hospitals by consulting with the patients' community pharmacist, one of every five admissions has been associated with a DRP, when all age groups are combined. Almost one-third of patients age 65 or older had DRPs that influenced their need for admission. Two-thirds of these problems were drug misuse, especially underuse of needed medications, and one-third of DRPs were adverse drug reactions and interactions to prescribed therapy taken as ordered. The most important factors (% of patients) associated with these problems were lack of patient knowledge of prescribed therapy (47.6), inability to afford the medication (32.3) and physician and pharmacist lack of knowledge that a DRP had influenced the patient's admission (88).[5]

Once in the hospital, almost one-third of patients over age 65 had an adverse reaction on the medical services in over 10,000 patients studied in 9 hospitals around the world, a rate which is slightly higher than the general hospital population.[6] A national sample of medication errors found that 12.2% and 11.0% of doses in nursing homes and hospitals, respectively, were given in error, with omission of needed doses and unauthorized drugs the preponderance of those serious drug misuse errors.[7]

Nursing Home Admissions and Length of Stay Problems

An average of three DRPs per patient was found on all consecutive admissions to a nursing home. Paradoxically, only one-third of the patients' total medical care problems had been identified before admission to the facility. Medication misuse, unnecessary therapy, therapy needed for newly identified problems, adverse drug reactions and missing lab and physical data needed to evaluate drug therapy were the most common DRPs noted on admission.[8] The DRPs identified were considered to be the cause of admission in over one-half (26 of 50) of the cases.

Once in the long term care facility, rigorous drug regimen reviews conducted monthly by regulatory mandate found significant DRPs of drug misuse and adverse reaction and interaction as well as contraindications to drug therapy (Tables 2 and 3) in 65% of cases.[9] The involuntary termination of these rigorous drug regimen review

TABLE 2. Adverse Drug Reactions and Interactions in a 72-Bed Nursing Home Over a 2-Year Period[15]

Drug Class(es)	Associated With Problem:		Number (%)	
Psychotropics Antipsychotics Anticonvulsants Antianxiety agents Antidepressants Sedative/Hypnotics Antihistamines and Opiate Analgesics	Pseudodementia or CNS depression which improved on discontinuance (D/C) or drugs(s) or lower dose	Single Drug Multiple Drugs Sub-Total	16 19 35	(21.7)
Antihypertensive Multiple Antihypertensive(s)	Low Blood Pressure Less than 110-120 mmHg 60-70 Which increased on D/C of drug or lower drug dose	Single Drug Multiple Drug Sub-Total	23 4 27	(16.8)
K-Wasting Diuretic with KCl Supplement	Hyperkalemia (K > 5. 0 mEq/L)		4	
K-Sparing Diuretic with KCl Supplement	Hyperkalemia (K > 5.0 mEq/L)		9	
K-Sparing Diuretic without KCl Supplement	Hyperkalemia (K > 5.0 mEq/L)		5	
		Sub-Total	18	(11.2)
K-Wasting Diuretic without KCl Supplement	Hypokalemia (K < 3.5 mEq/L)		11	
K-Wasting Diuretic with KCl Supplement	Hypokalemia (K < 3.5 mEq/L)	Sub-Total	2 13	
Digoxin Without Diuretic	Digoxin Toxicity Trough level > 2.0 ng/ml chronic weight (1-2 lbs/ month) loss—poor appetite or pulse < 60 BPM 3 or more times per month which improved on D/C or		12	
Digoxin Without Diuretic	lower dose drug		5	
		Sub-Total	17	(10.6)
Nonsteroidal Antiinflammatory Drugs (NSAIDs)	Gastrointestinal Bleeding, positive occult blood in stool and/or decreased hemoglobin/hematocrit	Single Drug Multiple NSAIDs	16 3	
		Sub-Total	19	(11.8)
Antacids with Methenamine, Tetra- cycline, Iron Salts, or Digoxin	Patient infection anemia or heart failure not improved or worsened	Sub-Total	8 8	(5.0)
Antiinfectives (Peni- cillins and sulfonamides)	Allergic Rash		8	(5.0)

Drug Class(es)	Associated With Problem:	Number (%)
Antidiabetics	FBS Less Than 60 mg/dL	5 (3.2)
KCI Liquid and Anti-infectives	Diarrhea	2 (1.2)
Psyllium Seed	Impactions due to insufficient oral fluids	1 (0.6) 1 (0.6)
Acetazolamide	Systemic Acidosis	1 (0.6)
Clindamycin	Pseudomembranous Colitis	1 (0.6)
Quinidine	Thrombocytopenic Purpura	1 (0.6)
Phenylbutazone/ Warfarin	GI ulcer perforation and massive intrabdom-inal hemorrhage (Protime rose from 21.4 to 61 seconds).	1 (0.6)
Opthalmic Dexa-methasone Drops (Continuous)	Glaucoma/Cataracts	1 (0.6)
Nitrofurantoin	Hemolytic anemia, improved on D/C	1 (0.6)
Nitrofurantoin	Pneumonitis, improved on D/C	1 (0.6)
L-DOPA/Pyridoxine	Worsening Parkinsonism	1 (0.6)
	Total	161 (100.0)

services has been associated with doubling of drugs per patient, increase in DRPs, and death rate. Subsequent re-initiation of these drug regimen reviews in the same facility has been found to lower admission, discharge, and death rates and cut drugs per patient in half.[10] In all three studies, the factors associated with DRPs were failure to adequately document patient problems and follow rational drug therapy principles, ignoring stated DRPs brought to the prescriber's attention, and lack of intensive diagnostic work-up and follow-up on the patients.[8,9,10]

Over a 4-year period, two-thirds of nursing facility residents had a mean of almost two probable adverse drug reactions.[11] The main factors in those who experienced an adverse drug reaction were polypharmacy (i.e., twice as many drugs as active problems) and failure to consider the history and total problem list of the patient. An adverse drug reaction-related hospitalization study of nursing facility patients has recently implicated NSAID gastropathy and psychotropic-associated fall injuries as the most common drug classes causing admissions.[12] A further study has documented that the pharmacist can decrease such NSAID-related hospitalizations by requesting monthly to bi-monthly hemoglobin and hematocrit

TABLE 3. Relative-to-Absolute Contraindications to Drug Usage Found in 2-Year Nursing Home Study[15]

Drug Class	Number	(%)	Preexisting Condition/ Diagnosis
Nonsteroidal Antiinflammatory Drugs (NSAID)	62	(30.7)	History of peptic ulcer disease with bleeding associated with NSAIDs
Potassium Chloride Supplements or Potassium Sparing Diuretics	48	(23.8)	History of moderate to severe* renal impairment
Tetracycline, Nalidixic acid, Nitrofurantoin or Methenamine Complexes	41	(20.3)	History of moderate to severe* renal impairment
Magnesium Containing Antacids or Milk of Magnesia	29	(14.4)	History of moderate to severe* renal impairment
Reserpine, Long acting Benzodiazepines, or Barbiturates	15	(7.3)	History/evidence of depression
Thiazide Diuretic	4	(2.0)	Creatinine clearance less than 10ml/min.
Digoxin	3	(1.5)	Second to third degree heart block, pulse less than 50
Total	202	(100.0)	

*Per W.M. Bennett, et al. Drug Prescribing in Renal Failure: Dosing Guidelines for Adults. Am.J. Kid. Dis., 1983: 5:155-193 (Reprints: The National Kidney Foundation, 2 Park Ave., New York, NY 10016, ($3.00)).

determinations and recommending alternative therapy when there is evidence of falling hematologic parameters or history of prior gastrointestinal problems from NSAID usage.[13]

In terms of drug-related falls and injuries within the nursing facility, alternative pharmacotherapy recommendations have been shown to reduce falls, fall-related fractures, hematomas and lacerations, pressure ulcers as well as emergency room and hospitalizations and patient fall costs by $177 to 197 per month by performing fall and psychoactive drug risk assessments and communication of recommendations to attending physicians.[14] In an earlier two-year study in this population, over 60% (98 of 161) of the adverse drug reactions (ADRs) were judged to be preventable by careful attention to the patients' complete history, problem list, and relative-to-absolute contraindications to the use of the drugs.[15] Forty-seven of the ADRs resulted in hospitalizations, at an average cost of $3,479 per episode. In a further study of 202 cases of contraindications to drug use that were taken into account in this same study population and period, the most common preexisting conditions/diagnoses taken into account to prevent ADRs are noted in Table 2.[16] Special drug considerations for appropriate drug usage in older patients are found in a prior review.[17]

The use of drugs in nursing homes has been recently reviewed.[18] This review focused on the development of specific criteria for inappropriate medications usage, the most common types of inappropriate prescribing, psychoactive drug use, antidepressants, pain and bowel function management and preventive aspects of falls, cardiovascular disease, infections, osteoporosis, and NSAID gastropathy.[18]

The "swing-bed" concept has been proposed as an alternative method of handling geriatric patient transition from the hospital to the nursing home. A study of swing-bed patients found that within a 20-day average length of stay, 65% had an adverse drug reaction, and 60% of patients exceeded their per diem total care allowance in drug costs alone, within the first 3 days of their swing-bed admission.[19] The apparent reasons for the DRPs noted were again incomplete work-up, failure to adequately monitor patient progress, "dumping" patients prematurely when all of their Medicare hospital days had been used up, and mismatching patients with this level of care.

Home Health and Day Care Patient Problems

Home health patients have significant DRPs of misuse in over one-half of cases evaluated. The most common DRPs were stopping or changing doses without professional consultation when the patient was on needed chronic care medication.[20] Similar findings were noted in an older adult day care study.[21] At both levels of care the apparent reasons for the problems were a lack of patient knowledge and comprehension of both disease states and pharmacotherapy, lack of thorough evaluation of patient status and therapeutic progress, and perceived lack of pharmacist and prescriber interest in the care of the patient.

Ambulatory Patient Problems

In a study of drug-related problems in a multiple-site ambulatory geriatric population, 53.4% of patients had significant DRPs. Misuse and adverse drug reaction were again the most common problems. Patient misperception of drug knowledge and prescriber and pharmacist lack of detection of drug-related problems by thorough drug regimen review were factors associated with these problems.[22]

It appears from existing drug-related problem studies, that problems of misuse and adverse reaction are quite common in the elderly at all levels of care.

III. TYPES OF DRUG-RELATED PROBLEMS AND ASSOCIATED FACTORS

Drug-related problems (DRPs) are of two main types: misuse (also termed noncompliance or nonadherence) and adverse drug reactions and interactions. Fully two-thirds of DRPs are misuse or non-compliance (approximately two-thirds of which are underuse and one-third are overuse) and adverse drug reactions and interactions account for the other third of DRPs in hospital, nursing home, home health, and day or self-care. The prevalence of DRPs influencing the need for hospital and nursing home admissions increases with age. When community and hospital pharmacists cooperate in obtaining a complete drug history on admission to small hospitals, one-fifth of patients across all age groups, but one-third of those 65 or over in a 500-patient study in two communities had a DRP that influenced their need for hospital admission. Non-compliance may be the most common drug-related problem seen influencing the need for hospital admission of elderly patients.[5]

Compliance is defined as adherence to prescribed or recommended therapy from one or more modalities of treatment and/or prevention; non-compliance is lack of adherence to therapy and/or preventive measures to the detriment of the patient.

Lack of compliance and care of oneself is not a recent problem—

> . . . As many as 7 of 10 persons who need my medical advice are the 'worried well' who don't follow my advice. . . . (Galen, ca. 129-199, C.E.)

... Keep watch also on the fault of patients which often make them lie about the taking of things prescribed. . . . (Hippocrates, ca. 460-370, B.C.E.)

Even more recently, a medical educator wrote ". . . In an era where when efficacious therapies exist or are being developed at a rapid rate, it is truly discouraging that one-half of patients for whom appropriate therapy is prescribed fail to receive full benefit through inadequate adherence to treatment. . . ."[23]

Factors in Drug-Related Problems

Key factors in the DRP-related admission of patients[5] were: 88% of cases were not recognized as DRPs on admission; 48% of those with DRP-related admissions could not answer three questions concerning their medications:

1. What is the name of each medicine you are taking?
2. How are you supposed to take your medication?
3. What is your medication supposed to do for you?

In terms of affording medical care, over one-third of patients with DRPs had to choose between food and needed chronic medication purchases. In terms of prevention and solutions–drug history between community and hospital pharmacists, prescriber and pharmacists' recognition of DRPs, reinforcement of patient education and follow-up was reduced to 1 of 20 DRP-related (from 1 of 5) hospital admissions within 5 years in one community.[5]

A study of nursing home admissions found that one-half of 50 consecutive admissions were associated with DRPs–most commonly medication non-compliance.[8] Again, the key factors were drug history, intensive drug regimen review by physicians and pharmacists. Only one-half of active problems were recognized prior to nursing home admission, especially malnutrition, anemia and depression.[8]

TYPES OF NON-COMPLIANCE

There are three main types of non-compliance according to usage patterns of non-compliance: underuse, overuse or erratic patterns of either overuse and/or underuse. There are also three types of non-compliance medication errors according to patient intent: unintentional, intentional and unintentional leading to intentional errors. Unintentional medication errors can be missed doses, wrong doses, drugs, time or schedule.

In the case of missed doses, when is this significant? If it is assumed, for example, that 80% of high blood pressure medications have to be taken for adequate control of blood pressure, but only 20-30% of patients are compliant, when thoroughly evaluated, then what is the effect on target organ damage to the eyes, heart, brain and kidney? In hospitals and nursing homes, some 10-12% of doses are subject to medication errors and omission of ordered doses is the most common medication error.[7] Wrong dose medication errors occur primarily because some liquids and injectable dosage forms are hard-to-measure, and ophthalmic solutions are commonly given in excessive dose. These constitute the most common sources of this type of error, which may be avoided by the use of total dosage from unit-of-use distribution systems. Wrong time errors occur when medications are given other than before, with, or after meals. Problems of reduced bioavailability to adverse drug reactions are common when this type of error occurs. Wrong schedule medication errors occur for example when a drug is given QID vs. q 6 h, or an after meals schedule with a patient who eats only one meal per day. Failure to remove transdermal nitroglycerin patches for 10-12 hours or to allow a sufficient nitrate-free interval and crushing sustained-release medications may also result in an improper schedule and either expose the patient to supra- or subtherapeutic drug levels. This leaves the patient at risk for both lack of therapeutic effect and increased toxicity.

Intentional medication errors are usually adverse drug reaction (ADR) and/or patient or caregiver-related disbelief or denial of illness-related omissions or abuse and overuse of psychoactive medications, such as benzodiazepines. Drug-abuse research indicates that up to one-seventh of the population are genetically and/or environmentally predisposed to abuse psychoactive drugs from alcohol to marihuana, cocaine, as well as "legitimate" but less than safe drugs such as the benzodiazepines and barbiturates.

Unintentional non-compliance can lead to intentional non-compliance. When a patient inadvertently skipped doses of a medication and note that they may feel better when they do not take the drug, the patient then purposely quits taking the drug. The sympatholytic antihypertensives are a class of drugs which are subject to this type of error.

Reasons for Patient Non-Compliance

1. Lack of patient knowledge of disease and drugs;
2. Patient disbelief or denial of illness and distrust of health care;
3. Cost of medications and having to choose between purchasing drugs or other life necessities (e.g., food);
4. Complexity of regimen–especially when more than 3 drugs and 6 to 10 doses per day are required to comply;
5. Lack of patient activation and interest in their health maintenance and/or knowledge of "Wellness" or self-care concepts;
6. Lack of comprehensive drug regimen review and compliance assessment;
7. Patient may feel worse taking than not taking drug;
8. Unacceptable risk/benefit for drug usage;
9. Willful abuse of drugs;
10. Health care provider attitudes toward medications;
11. Lack of continuity of care between levels of care;
12. Lack of communication between health care providers.

Issues for Consideration in Compliance and Preventive Care

"High touch and low tech" may be the best way to care for patients. The recent report of the U.S. Preventive Service Task Force[23] data shows that efforts made by clinicians to influence health behaviors are more likely to reduce morbidity and mortality than any other clinical intervention.

We are in the process of changing the way health care is financed from crisis-dominated to wellness awareness and prevention under managed care. Third-party financed, managed health care is a reality, but the elderly may not get as good a quality of care when compared to fee-for-service systems.[4] Crisis health care payment on the other hand with a "blank check" approach to financing is history. Diagnosis-related groups (DRGs) methods of payment in hospitals may be applied to community care; vertical integration of levels of care and horizontal proliferation with ill-defined boundaries is now present.

IV. UNDERRECOGNITION OF PROBLEMS OF THE ELDERLY

In the community-at-large many health and aging-related problems that go underrecognized include: depression, sensory changes in sight, taste, touch and hearing, osteoarthritis, cardiovascular problems of high blood pressure and ischemic heart disease and strokes, and malnutrition.[2,8]

On admission to long-term care facilities or nursing homes the most commonly underrecognized and undertreated problems are malnutrition, depression, sensory deficits, anemia, osteoporosis and pressure ulcers.[8] During the nursing home stay the most commonly undertreated problems are high blood pressure, chronic constipation, chronic urinary tract infection, osteoarthritis, depression, glaucoma, angina pectoris, seizures, transient ischemic attacks and malnutrition.[8]

V. MISDIAGNOSIS OF PROBLEMS OF THE ELDERLY

One study has shown that there can be significant diagnostic discrepancies on nursing home admission. Almost two-thirds of admission diagnoses were inaccurate, primarily labeling patients with dementia, when depression was the problem, chronic seizure disorder when only one seizure had occurred after a stroke.[25]

VI. PHARMACEUTICAL INDUSTRY AND REGULATORY PERSPECTIVES

There has been much improvement in the way that the pharmaceutical industry stereotypes elderly patients in an attempt to influence prescribing habits. The tragedy of drugs like benoxaprofen, longer-acting benzodiazepines and non-steroidal antiinflammatories associated respectively with increased rates of falls and fractures and gastrointestinal bleeding has brought significant regulatory changes in the ways that new drugs could be approved.

The U.S. Food and Drug Administration (FDA) has recently conducted a review of post-approval risks of drugs released from 1976-1985. The FDA found that of the 198 drugs approved during this period, 51.5% had serious postapproval risks and many problems did not become evident until 5 or more years after the drug appeared on the market.[26]

A "guideline for the study of drugs likely to be used in the elderly" was issued by the FDA in 1989 to encourage routine and thorough evaluation of the effects of drugs in elderly populations.[27] The Omnibus Budget Reconciliation Act of 1987 (OBRA) and the Combined version (COBRA) of 1990 require reform in the way drugs are used in nursing home patients. A special concern for central nervous system drugs and antipsychotic drugs in particular requires that their usage be justified, that drugs NOT be used as chemical restraints as well as monitored daily for beneficial as well as adverse effects. The OBRA/COBRA also requires that the patients be free from "unnecessary drugs," and that detailed documentation on patients' conditions is mandated.[28]

Perhaps the most sweeping legislation affecting drug therapy in older adults in America is the 1993 Medicaid (i.e., primarily state-funded medications for geriatric patients) requirement that all patients receive patient counseling, that prospective drug regimen review be conducted when each new prescription is written, and that adverse drug reactions and poor compliance be detected and communicated by the community pharmacist to patient and the prescriber.[29] If estimated costs of non-compliance and adverse drug reactions are 16-20 billion dollars per year to the American health care system, there is considerable potential for cost savings.[23]

A recent report on drug misuse among the American homebound elderly (95% of those over 65 years of age) demonstrated that it is not always the patient or prescriber making dosage errors. More than one-half of the caregivers of dependent or frail elderly have responsibility for administering and monitoring medications, and often don't understand the drugs or the regimen. A U.S. Inspector

General's report showed that although those over 60 make up only 17% of the American population, they represent 39% of all hospitalizations and 51% of the deaths from drug reactions. This report noted that in 1987 at least 200,000 older adults were hospitalized due to an adverse drug reaction, or experienced an ADR while hospitalized. The recommendations of this report are detailed elsewhere.[24,26,27,30]

The Institute of Medicine of the National Academy of Sciences recently recommended from a workshop on drug development for the geriatric population the following:

1. design drugs specifically for the elderly;
2. when evaluating geriatric drugs, consider the patients' ability to function normally, not just the drugs' efficacy and side effects;
3. consider the possible negative effects of drug cost "caps" when designing drug policy;
4. include persons over age 85 in drug studies;
5. develop methods for disseminating research findings to physicians; and
6. develop more training programs in geriatric medicine.[30]

The Pharmaceutical Manufacturers Association (PMA) in its third annual survey of new medicines in development for older Americans showed that 329 medicines are in development for 45 diseases that commonly affect older people.[31]

VII. TOUGH CHOICES IN A WORLD OF SHRINKING RESOURCES

Simply decreasing the number of drugs per patient is not enough, however. In a study of 440 New Hampshire Medicaid recipients whose prescriptions were limited to 3 per month, the nursing home and hospital admission rates almost doubled.[32]

Daniel Callahan, Director of the Hastings Center and author of the book "Setting Limits" has proposed that the U.S. control health care expenditures, even if it means rationing care by age. It seems ludicrous he maintains that we ". . . spend the same 6 per cent of the

Gross National Product (GNP) on education that we did 30 years ago, but have almost doubled the cost of health care from 6 to 12% of the GNP. We are not investing as we should in education, basic infrastructure, manufacturing, research and development. It is also bizarre, that we have an inefficient health care system costing us more money while depriving more people of decent health care. We spend three times more on health care per capita than Britain . . . yet our outcomes are no better. . . ."[33] Differences in drug utilization per older patient are hard to understand: comparing the American with the British older adult, one finds that the average drug use per patient is 6 for Americans and 3 for the British, with no perceived difference in therapeutic outcome.[33]

VIII. GERIATRIC DISEASE MANAGEMENT

The concept of pharmaceutical care espouses a paradigm shift in which the pharmacist actually accepts responsibility for pharmacotherapeutic outcomes in patient care.[34] Within the nursing home setting it has been found that up to three-fourths of patients on digoxin can have the drug stopped, as they did not have chronic congestive heart failure. Up to 40% of hypertensive patients admitted to nursing homes may have their drugs stopped, as they do not have chronic hypertension. Up to 90% of antibiotics ordered for the urinary tract were for colonizations not infections, as the routine usage of urinalyses in incontinent patients commonly finds protective colonization of the bladder. Virtually all patients have some aspect of malnutrition. Over two-thirds of antipsychotics can be stopped in dementia patients. Over 80% of H-2 blocker drugs are given for excessive dosages and periods of therapy.[35,36]

Academicians face the responsibility for the education and evaluation to accomplish these outcomes, both before and after graduation. Professional associations provide a base for the sustained growth, political voice and sophistication of their members. Regulatory agencies ensure compliance with a standard established by the profession. Reimbursement agencies juggle the overall cost of health care and depend on the strength of leadership and demonstration of competent cost-effective care by all practitioners, as well as search for every cost-savings measure that can be identified.[35,36,37]

Assumptions for Geriatric Drug Therapy Interventions Research

1. Before any health care provider can assume responsibility for pharmacotherapy outcomes in health care, there has to be a process of identification of those outcomes which are jointly affected by all health care practitioners. For example what are the current outcomes in terms of patient health care access and availability to primary care, compliance with all modalities of treatment as well as adoption of sound wellness and self-care measures, and drug effects on disease morbidity and mortality. Tables 4 and 5 list outcomes that should be primary or shared responsibilities of pharmacists with other health care providers.

2. Once the most important outcome measures have been identified, a prioritization of which outcomes can be most easily affected in one's practice area, state or region, whether or not there is com-

TABLE 4. Clinical Outcomes and Associated Processes

Outcome	Process(es)
Primary Pharmacist Responsibility	
Changes in:	
Drugs Per Patient	Intensive Drug Regimen Review (DRR)*
Fewer doses per patient per day	Intensive DRR
Improved compliance	Patient history, DRR, education of patient and their caregivers
Decreased adverse drug reactions and interactions	(same as compliance)
Decreased drug therapy-related emergency room visits	(same as compliance)
Decreased physician office visits and hospitalizations	(same plus patient assessment)
Decreased primary care costs for self-limited illness	(same plus patient assessment)
Shared Responsibility in Consultation with Other Health Care Providers	
Less expensive therapeutic alternatives	Patient assessment, DRR, and education plus pharmacotherapeutic consultation
Less expensive chronic disease management	(same as above)

*This may mean either an increase or decrease in medications

TABLE 5. Some Disease Specific Clinical Outcomes That May Be Shared by Pharmacist Contributions to Pharmacotherapy

Disease	Desirable Outcomes
Cardiovascular and high blood pressure	decreased myocardial infarctions (MIs), strokes, prolonged survival in heart failure and life-threatening arrhythmias as well as all complications
Angina Pectoris	Fewer MIs, anginal attacks, delayed complications
Peripheral Vascular Disease	Better circulation, fewer ulcers, decreased surgeries/amputations
COPD	Fewer acute attacks, infections, decreased hospitalizations
Diabetes Mellitus	Fewer hypoglycemic episodes, complications and hospitalizations
Acute and Chronic UTIs	Fewer Catheterizations, acute UTIs, less urosepsis
Incontinence	Bladder retraining, less constipation, fewer UTIs
Dementia	Improved psychotropic usage, fewer falls and fractures, agitation episodes and fewer insidious ADRs
Depression	Improved assessment, antidepressant usage, improved activities of daily living (ADLs) and socialization
Peptic Ulcer Disease	Fewer GI bleeds, and better chronic prevention
Osteoporosis	Fewer fractures and hip-nailing procedures
Renal Disease	Fewer ADRs due to inappropriate drug usage and slowing loss of function

plete agreement and support from other health care practitioners, can be formulated. Prior reviews have anecdotally established the most important drug-related problems are patient non-compliance and preventable adverse drug reactions and interactions.[35,36,37] Other health care practitioners are affected by any process pharmacy uses to lessen the frequency of these problems. While these interdisciplinary considerations are important, they should not impede progress by pharmacists to affect these outcomes.

3. There is no current profession-derived "standard of pharmaceutical care." There are a variety of reasons for this assumption. Even though all professional associations have codes of ethics, conduct, statements of principles or qualifications, there is no current statement to my knowledge that addresses a "standard of care" across all areas of professional involvement with patients: community, long-term care and hospital. Perhaps clinical outcomes research findings will help to provide a basis for such a standard.

4. There are at least two current regulatory agency-derived national mandates for pharmacists to provide clinical services: the 1974[38] and 1980 Federal requirement for monthly drug regimen review of the long term care patient, and the 1987 and 1990 Omnibus Budget Reconciliation Acts (OBRA) that require drug history, patient records and prospective drug regimen review as well as patient education.[28,29]

5. Pharmacists should be reimbursed for cognitive clinical services that prevent patient drug-related problems or improve the quality of care with medications if they are to survive as a health care practitioner. A corollary to this assumption is that the current system that pays for what is "filled" has to be changed to a system that combines payment more for service regardless of whether a drug is dispensed or not.

6. Pharmacy should formulate an action plan for clinical services and reimbursement in drug store, nursing home, home care or hospital practice settings.

Clinical activities of the pharmacist can be viewed as a continuum of effort from the time the patient enters ones' practice, whether in the community pharmacy, nursing home (facility), home health agency, hospital through periodic evaluations and subsequent "continuous" pharmacy care.[39]

Clinical activities may include:

1. A Complete Drug History.*
2. Developing a Problem List.
3. Establishing and Observing Physical and Laboratory Parameters for the Patient.

4. Patient-Oriented Medication Regimen Review.*
5. Communication of Clinically Significant Problems.*
6. Adverse Drug Reactions, Anticipation Prevention, and Recognition.*
7. Patient Care Rounds and Conferences.
8. Pharmacokinetic, Therapeutic and Nutritional Consultations.
9. Medication Regimen Compliance by Patient, Family, Prescriber, Nursing, and Aide Personnel.
10. Patient, Family, Prescriber and Caregiver Education.*
11. Provision of Objective Drug Information, Retrieval, Analysis and Communications.
12. Primary Care Activities of the Consultant Pharmacist.*
    * = Required by OBRA as of January, 1993[28]

Primary care by the pharmacist in long-term care facilities is the most recent clinical activity of the consultant. The State of California currently has changed its regulations to allow pharmacists with doctoral level training to provide primary care under physician supervision to nursing home patients. The results of this study were a savings of $70,000 per year per 100 nursing home beds.[40] In terms of specific disease states, the pharmacist has been shown to improve therapeutic outcomes in diabetes mellitus,[41] high blood pressure,[42] COPD,[43] and depression.[44]

Some improved therapeutic outcomes that may be evident from pharmacist involvement in disease state management are listed in Table 5.

There are a number of valid research questions and recommendations for interventions in geriatric drug therapy care to be raised from this review:

1. Why are drug-related problems so prevalent at all levels of care? Should larger-scale studies be done, utilizing similar rigorous methods to identify, quantify and find methods to reduce this prevalence?
2. What are the educational, socioeconomic, psychological and quality of medical care ramifications of drug-related problems and disease state management by the pharmacist?

3. What interventions are most cost-effective in identification and reduction of drug-related problems and improved disease state management?
4. What funding initiatives should be encouraged from private and public groups that should be responsive to these issues?
5. How can health care practitioners work together to identify and reduce drug-related problems and disease state management in their respective practices?
6. How can elderly health care consumers become more aware of the magnitude of drug-related problems and more active in their own preventive self-care and disease state management?

As Benjamin Disraeli stated, ". . . the health of the nation is the foundation upon which their happiness depends. . . ." In terms of pharmacist intervention in health care of the geriatric patient, a medical educator has remarked that the pharmacist interface at the use if drugs by patients is needed and ". . . in the long run, in medical care as well as all other areas of human endeavor in a free society, whoever is available at the right time to do a necessary job best, fastest, and cheapest will get and keep that job."[45]

REFERENCES

1. Anonymous. McKnight's Long Term Care News, July 1990.
2. Schneider EL, Guralnik JM. The aging of America: impact on health care costs. JAMA 1990;263:2335-2340.
3. US Department of Health, Education and Welfare. PHSRA. Pharmacy and the elderly. Center for Human Services, 1979. DHEW publication no. (HRA) 80-36 and 37.
4. Ware JE, Bayliss MS, Rogers WH et al. Differences in 4-year health outcomes for elderly and poor chronically ill patients treated in HMO and fee-for-service systems. JAMA 1996;276:1039-1047.
5. Frisk PA, Cooper JW, Campbell NA. Community-hospital pharmacist detection of drug-related problems upon patient admission to small hospitals. Am J Hosp Pharm 1977; 34:738-742.
6. Miller RR. Drug surveillance utilizing epidemiologic methods–a report from the Boston Collaborative Drug Surveillance Program. Am J Hosp Pharm 1973; 30: 584-592.
7. Barker KN, Mikeal RL, Pearson RE et al. Medication errors in nursing homes and small hospitals. Am J Hosp Pharm 1982; 39:987-991.
8. Cooper JW. Effects of intensive consultant pharmacy review of nursing home admission orders. Cons Pharm 1987; 2:152-155.

9. Cooper JW. Drug-related problems in geriatric nursing home patients. J Ger Drug Ther 1986; 1(1):47-68.

10. Cooper JW. Effect of initiation, termination, and re-initiation of consultant clinical pharmacist services in a geriatric long-term care facility. Med Care 1985; 23:84-88.

11. Cooper JW. Probable adverse drug reactions in a rural geriatric nursing home population: a four-year study. J Am Geriatr Soc 1996;44:194-197.

12. Cooper JW. Adverse drug reaction-related hospitalizations of nursing home patients: a four-year study, submitted.

13. Cooper JW. Consultant pharmacist effect on NSAID-related hospitalizations of nursing facility residents, submitted.

14. Cooper JW, Cobb HH. Buspirone conversion of nursing facility patients with falls and fall-related injuries, submitted.

15. Cooper JW. Adverse drug reactions and interactions in a nursing home. Nursing Homes 1987; 36(4): 7-11.

16. Cooper JW. Drug-related problems in nursing home patients: Contraindications to drug usage. Nursing Homes 1987; 36(3): 5-7.

17. Cooper JW. Reviewing geriatric concerns with commonly used drugs. Geriatrics 1989; 44(oct):79-86.

18. Avorn J, Gurwitz JH. Drug use in nursing homes. Ann Intern Med 1995;123:195-204.

19. Cooper JW. Drug-related problems in swing-bed patients. Cons Pharm 1988; 3: 257.

20. Cooper JW, Griffin DL, Francisco GE et al. Home-health Care: drug-related problems detected by consultant pharmacist participation. Hosp Form 1985; 20:643-650.

21. Cooper JW. Drug-related problems in day-care patients. Cons Pharm 1988; 3: 193.

22. Wade WE, Cobb HH, Cooper JW. Drug-related problems in a multiple site ambulatory geriatric population. J Ger Drug Ther 1986; 1(2):67-79.

23. Eraker SA et al. Non-compliance in older adults. Ann Int Med 1984; 100:258-68.

24. Contemp Senior Health Vol.1, No.1 Summer 1989, "Guide to Preventive Clinical Services."

25. Miller JA et al. Diagnostic errors on nursing home admission. JAGS 1977;25:108.

26. FDA Drug review: postapproval risks 1976-1985. GAO PO Box 6015, Gaithersburg, MD 20877.

27. FDA Guideline for the study of drugs likely to be used in the elderly. J Geratri Drug Ther 1990; 5(2): 5-18.

28. Omnibus Budget Reconciliation Act of 1987 and Combined revision of 1990, U.S. Congress, Public Law 100-203.

29. 1993 Amendment to the Social Security Act, Title XVIII and XIX, U.S. Congress.

30. Drug development for the geriatric population. Institute of Medicine, National Academy of Sciences, 2101 Constitution Ave., NW, Washington, DC 20418.

31. Anonymous. Consultant Pharm. 1991:6(10):858.

32. Anonymous. McKnight's Long Term Care News. August 1990.

33. Anonymous. ASCP Update August 1990.

34. Hepler CD, Strand LM. Opportunities and responsibilities in pharmaceutical care. Am J Pharm Ed 1989; 53:7S-15S.

35. Cooper JW. Cost-Savings: The Value of the Pharmacist Consultant. J Pharm Pract. 1988; 1:173-7.

36. Cooper JW. Consultant Pharmacist Impact on Health Care in America. The Consult Pharm, 1988; 3:342-6.

37. Cooper JW. Drug Related Problems in Geriatric Nursing Home Patients. Binghamton, NY: The Haworth Press, Inc., 1991.

38. Federal Register, January 17, 1974; 228.

39. Cooper JW, Frisk PA, Walchle RC. Continuous Clinical Pharmacy Care–A Method to Reduce Drug-Related Problems in the Small Community. J Clin Pharmacol, 1975; 15: 55.

40. Thompson JF, McGhan WF, Ruffalo JT et al. Clinical Pharmacists Prescribing Drug Therapy in a Skilled-Nursing Facility: Outcome of a Trial. J Am Geriatr Soc 1984; 32:154-9.

41. Cooper JW. Consultant pharmacist contribution to diabetes mellitus treatment outcomes in two patient outcomes in two nursing facilities. Cons Pharm 1995; 10(1):13-18.

42. Skaer TL et al. Effect of value-added utilities on prescription refill compliance and health care expenditures for hypertension. J Hum Hyperten 1993; 7(5):515-518.

43. Sclar DA et al. Ipatropium in the management of chronic obstructive pulmonary disease: effect on health service expenditures. Clin Ther 1994; 16(4):595-601.

44. Sclar DA et al. Antidepressant pharmacotherapy: economic outcomes in a health maintenance organization. Clin Ther 1994; 16(4):715-730.

45. Lundberg GD, Editorial. JAMA 1983;249:1193.

RESEARCH ARTICLES

Documentation
of Pharmacists' Interventions
in the Ambulatory Setting:
Results with Geriatric Patients

Jack E. Fincham
Jacqueline B. Hunter

SUMMARY. A sample of twenty-five community pharmacies was selected to serve as study sites for a project designed to document the worth of pharmacist interventions in patients' drug therapy. A total of 709 interventions were reported during a four week data collection period. Study pharmacists recorded their intervention activities on a one page data collection form. Of the interventions reported, a total of 212 (30%) were made with geriatric patients.

Jack E. Fincham, PhD, is Dean and Professor of Pharmacy Practice, The University of Kansas School of Pharmacy, Lawrence, KS 66045. Jacqueline B. Hunter, BS PharmD, was a student at the time of the study and is now affiliated with the Creighton University School of Pharmacy, Omaha, NE 68178.

This proposal was funded by the NARD Foundation/SmithKline Beecham Consumer Healthcare Research Grant Program.

[Haworth co-indexing entry note]: "Documentation of Pharmacists' Interventions in the Ambulatory Setting: Results with Geriatric Patients." Fincham, Jack E., and Jacqueline B. Hunter. Co-published simultaneously in *Journal of Geriatric Drug Therapy* (The Pharmaceutical Products Press, an imprint of The Haworth Press, Inc.) Vol. 11, No. 4, 1997, pp. 27-42; and: *Geriatric Drug Therapy Interventions* (ed: James W. Cooper) The Pharmaceutical Products Press, an imprint of The Haworth Press, Inc., 1997, pp. 27-42. Single or multiple copies of this article are available for a fee from The Haworth Document Delivery Service [1-800-342-9678, 9:00 a.m. - 5:00 p.m. (EST). E-mail address: getinfo@haworth.com].

Direct savings due to the actions of the pharmacist amount to an average of $20.20 for each of the generic substitutions, $35.36 for therapeutic substitutions, $28.82 for drug discontinuances, and $46.32 for drugs deemed not necessary to dispense. Indirect costs saved for avoidance of hospitalization, emergency room visits, and physician office visits were estimated to total $137,505 for the geriatric patients for the study period. This amounted to $1,297 in avoided outcome costs for each of the applicable interventions. By extrapolating the data for an entire year, the resultant savings to the health care system through pharmacists' interventions in these twenty-five pharmacies would amount to $1,787,565 for geriatric patients alone.

The data collected through this study are indicative of the breadth and depth of pharmacist activities in the community pharmacy practice setting which save enormous amounts of expenditures for medical care to treat potential adverse drug-related sequelae in geriatric patients. In addition to economic savings, the actions of the pharmacists were shown to enhance the appropriate use, discontinuance, or avoidance of certain drug therapies which in turn enhanced the quality of pharmaceutical care of the patients affected. Pharmacists deserve to be paid for such interventions which avert the spending of unnecessary health care dollars. *[Article copies available for a fee from The Haworth Document Delivery Service: 1-800-342-9678. E-mail address: getinfo@haworth.com]*

KEYWORDS: pharmacists, interventions, ambulatory, geriatric

INTRODUCTION

Pharmacists perform countless activities that save time and money, benefit patients and physicians, save third party payers money, and enhance the delivery of health care services. Yet, the impact of pharmacist intervention in drug therapies is increasingly in need of documentation. The purpose of this study was to collect data regarding the benefits of interventions by community pharmacists, analyze the cost savings associated with the intervention, propose a framework for pharmacists to use to collect and analyze such data, and work to develop a mechanism to document such activities so as to be reimbursed for such activities by third party payers.

The benefits of interventions by pharmacists have been described in the literature of pharmacy. Recently, more and more articles have appeared which indicate the cost savings associated with the efforts of pharmacists to intervene in drug therapy. These studies indicate an enhanced quality of life for patients, and an improved profit potential for the pharmacy.[1] Pharmacists routinely perform activities that result in economic and therapeutic benefits to patients and third party payers. In one large-scale study, it was noted that roughly 2% of prescriptions examined had one or more prescribing errors.[2] In other studies, diaries have been suggested to be used to quantify and record the interventions that pharmacists routinely make.[3] Elsewhere, the influence of pharmacists has produced lower drug expenditures, and in some cases the administration of fewer doses.[4] In managed care settings, the interventions of pharmacists have been calculated to be $24.00 per intervention.[5] Other interventions have been suggested to be included in these cost benefit, or cost effectiveness assessments. For example, patient counseling and patient compliance have been targeted to be included in future economic determinations.[6] Cost avoidance assessments have also been suggested to be included in these type of impact studies.[7,8] Managed care settings currently collect and analyze such data.[9] Recently, a group of researchers in Washington State have developed a framework to collect some data, and seek to obtain reimbursement for such activities for pharmacists performing cognitive service activities. Excluded items in their framework, however, include patient counseling, and compliance monitoring.[10]

The project results described in this report build upon a previous NARD Foundation sponsored project which indicated that pharmacists' interventions improved clinical, economic, and humanistic outcomes.[11] These types of analyses are important to the structuring of a means to gather such data in the community pharmacy setting, analyze the cost-benefit, and cost-effectiveness properties of these interventions, and determine how the data can best be collected on a larger scale for ease in assessing the economic worth of the interventions. The ultimate goal is to document the worth of interventions, and subsequently have pharmacists reimbursed for such efforts.

METHODS

A convenience sample of thirty pharmacies in both rural (population less than 25,000) and urban areas throughout Kansas was selected to carry out the study. The thirty pharmacists were contacted by letter and/or phone, and all accepted the invitation to participate. The pharmacies included in the sample were selected from urban and rural strata so as to gain a complete cross-sectional profile of community pharmacy practice in the U.S. Twenty-five pharmacies actually participated in the study. The remaining five pharmacies chose not to participate for various reasons. Pharmacists were requested to collect data for a four week period of time. A data collection form was designed to capture data detailing a pharmacist intervention in a patient's drug therapy. A sample data collection form can be found in Appendix A. Data collection forms were sent to each pharmacist prior to the study initiation. Accompanying the forms was an instruction sheet describing how the form should be completed. Please see Appendix B for a copy of the instruction sheet. At the bottom of the form a phone number for the project directors was also listed for participants to contact the study director if necessary.

The pharmacists were to describe their own interventions, document the activities that they implemented to deal with the identified problem, and estimate the cost savings associated with their activities. Other studies have utilized observers of pharmacist intervention activities.[12]

RESULTS

A total of twenty-five of the thirty project pharmacies forwarded interventions for analysis. A total of 709 interventions were forwarded to the study directors for analysis; of this number, 212 (29%) involved geriatric patients.

Prescription Status, and Prescription Source

Concerning the prescription status of the interventions, 129 (60.7%) were for new prescriptions, 19 (10.3%) were for refill prescriptions, and 32 (17.3%) were for over-the-counter drugs (OTCs). The patient was the source for 158 of the intervention prescriptions (90.8%), and a doctor phoned in prescription was the source for 11 (6.3%) of the intervention prescriptions.

Patient Demographics

Several types of demographic data were collected via the intervention sheets (age and gender).

Gender. A total of 131 (62.7%) of the intervention patients were female, 78 (37.3%) were male, and for 3 (1.4%) of the interventions gender was not reported.

Age. The mean age of geriatric patients for whom interventions were reported was 72.9 years, S.D. 8.54, range 60-97 years. The mode of the sample was 65 years.

Reason for Intervention

There were four possible categories of reasons (with varying response subheadings under each category) for pharmacist interventions (prescribing errors–5 options, prescription omission–7 options, drug therapy monitoring–7 options, and drug interactions–5 options). Please see Appendix A for a copy of the intervention form. Pharmacist participants could check any and all of the potential twenty-four reasons for intervention options.

Located in Table 1 are the intervention types classified as prescribing errors by the study participants. A total of 51 of the interventions were classified as prescribing errors. The reason of "inappropriate dose/regimen/strength" was the largest category checked in this grouping.

TABLE 1. Prescribing Error Interventions

Reason	Frequency
1. Inappropriate Drug/Indication	14
2. Inappropriate Dose/Regimen/Strength	28
3. Inappropriate Dosage Form	4
4. Inappropriate Quantity/Duration	3
5. Incorrect Patient	2
Total	51

Located in Table 2 are the intervention types classified as drug therapy monitoring by the study participants. A total of 157 of the interventions were classified as drug therapy monitoring interventions.

Located in Table 3 are the intervention types classified as prescription omissions. A total of 32 of the interventions were classified as prescription omissions.

Located in Table 4 are the intervention types classified as drug interactions. A total of 37 interventions were listed as drug interactions. Drug interactions occurring between two or more prescription drugs were the major reason for interventions in this grouping (21 interventions), followed by prescription and OTC products (7 interventions).

The drugs identified by the pharmacists that were involved in the interventions can be found listed in Appendix C. As can be determined by review of the drugs involved, agents included in analgesic, gastrointestinal, anti-infective, NSAID, muscle relaxant, headache medication, hyperlipidemic, ophthalmic, antiepileptic, home care product, benzodiazepine, antidepressant, psychotropic, topical, antidiabetic, cardiovascular, sex hormone, adrenal

TABLE 2. Drug Therapy Monitoring Interventions

Reason	Frequency
1. Side effects/toxicity/allergic reactions	20
2. Duplicate therapy	8
3. Overutilization	24
4. Underutilization	10
5. Patient concern/question	49
6. Patient counseling	36
7. Compliance intervention	19
Total	157

TABLE 3. Prescription Omission Interventions

Reason	Frequency
1. Drug not specified	0
2. Dose/Regimen not specified	5
3. Form/Strength not specified/Unavailable	9
4. Quantity/Duration not specified	2
5. Incomplete directions for use	9
6. Illegible	4
7. Violates legal requirement	3
Total	32

TABLE 4. Drug Interactions Interventions

Type	Frequency
1. Prescription and over-the-counter	7
2. Prescription–Prescription	21
3. Allergy/sensitivity	2
4. Drug–Disease	1
5. Other	6
Total	37

corticosteroid, nutritional supplement, antiasthmatics/respiratory tract, antiemetic/antivertigo, weight loss product, and miscellaneous categories are represented in the listing of drugs.

Prescription Outcomes

Listed in Table 5 are the prescription outcomes of the interventions. In 21 of the interventions, the prescription was dispensed as written. In 53 of the interventions, the prescription order was clarified. In 14 of the intervention situations, the prescription was not dispensed. In 93 of the interventions, the order was changed and an item dispensed.

Direct Intervention Time

Listed in Table 6 are the values for the intervention times for the pharmacists' activities. The direct contact time spent during the intervention by the pharmacist with either the patient or patient representative, or other (prescriber, profile review or research) was not lengthy. The vast majority of contacts with either of the category sources was minimal (mean = 6.9 for patient representative, 7.46 for prescriber).

Therapeutic Outcome Avoided

The pharmacists were asked to indicate one or more of three therapeutic outcomes which were avoided by their intervention activ-

TABLE 5. Prescription Outcomes

Outcome	Frequency
1. Prescription dispensed as written	21
2. Prescription clarified and dispensed	53
3. Prescription changed and dispensed	93
4. Prescription not dispensed	14
Total	181

TABLE 6. Direct Intervention Time

Pharmacist contact time with?	Mean Time Spent in Minutes
Patient or patient representative, N = 147	7.46, S.D. 10.8, range 1-90
Other (prescriber, profile review, research), N = 155	6.9, S.D. 10.4, range 1-90

ities for each of the interventions. The three outcomes were emergency room visits, physician visits, and hospitalizations. Please see Table 7 for a description of the indirect cost avoidance outcomes of the interventions. The estimated cost savings for a physician visit was $75.00 per visit. This figure was derived as the average cost of a physician's office visit in the State of Kansas.[13] The average cost of an emergency room visit was estimated to be $474.00 based upon average rates of hospital costs for the West-North Central Region of the United States for state and local government hospitals plus physician service in the hospital.[14] The hospital costs were determined from the average costs associated with the average length of hospital stay and associated costs for the five DRG classifications 447-451 that deal with allergic reactions and/or toxic effects of drugs.[15] The amount used to represent the associated costs of each of the hospitalizations averted was $5,025.00. This method of cost determination had been previously used to determine average costs of hospital care.[12] The total estimated costs attributed to the pharmacists' interventions was $137,505. This breaks down to $1,297 per intervention for the 106 interventions where the pharmacist indicated that a therapeutic outcome was avoided. By extrapolating the data for an entire year, the resultant savings to the health care system through pharmacists' interventions in these pharmacies alone would amount to $1,787,565 for geriatric patients alone.

Drug Related Costs Saved

Drug related cost savings include generic substitution savings, therapeutic substitution savings, drug discontinuance savings, and savings accrued to a drug not being dispensed. The study pharmacists performed a total of 28 generic substitutions with an average savings of $20.19 (range, $2.02-$75.00). The pharmacists performed approved therapeutic substitutions saving $35.63 (range, $0.90-$90.00) for each of the 12 intervention classes of drugs affected. There were five drugs discontinued as a part of the pharmacist interventions, these discontinuances averaged $28.82 (range, $4.99-$70.00) per intervention. There were 6 drugs that were not dispensed for an average savings of $46.32 per prescription.

TABLE 7. Possible Therapeutic Outcome Avoided

Outcome	Frequency	Cost Avoided
1. Emergency Room Visit	24	$474.00 each
2. Physician Visit	52	$75.00 each
3. Hospitalization	4	$5,025.00 each
Outcomes 1, 2 and 3	10	$5,574.00 each
Outcomes 1 and 3	3	$5,499.00 each
Outcomes 1 and 2	8	$549.00 each
Outcomes 2 and 3	5	$5,100.00 each
	Total 106	Total Savings $137,505.00

DISCUSSION

The data collection form utilized for this study appeared to be easily completed by the pharmacist participants. The submitted forms were reviewed as they were received in order to uncover possible difficulties in completing the forms. The majority of forms were completed satisfactorily. No doubt, greater care would have been taken in completing the forms and the problem minimized if they were actually going to be submitted for reimbursement.

What appears to have influenced reporting was remembering to document many activities that pharmacists consider to be routine responsibilities of pharmacy practice. For example, several pharmacists indicated that patient counseling activities are now mandated by law and/or regulation, and because of this, only extraordinary counseling above and beyond the norm was listed as an intervention. Another routine activity that may have been underreported was generic substitution. This activity, although routinely performed, saves countless sums of money year in and year out.

The vast majority of identified interventions involved drug therapy monitoring. The identification of side effects, toxicity, or allergic reactions and subsequent counseling was the most commonly identified monitoring activity. Apart from therapy monitoring, a sizable number of interventions involved in identification and resolution of frank prescribing errors on the part of physicians and other prescribers was noted. The identification of drug interaction interventions was also a frequently noted activity.

The therapeutic outcomes which were listed due to the pharmacist interventions were estimated avoided occurrences which were determined by the pharmacist. There was not a validation procedure in the study to ensure that these estimated therapeutic avoidances were plausible. Nevertheless, the severity of the avoided outcome is apparent in many of the cases (e.g., prescribing of penicillin for a patient allergic to penicillin or over- or underutilization of antihypertensives). Based upon the findings of this study, as well as others, it may be useful to design a standardized method of cost savings attributable to a pharmacist intervention for geriatric as well as other populations. Through such a standardized method of estimating cost savings or cost minimization activities, it would be feasible to make a strong case to third party payers and others of the worth and need to compensate pharmacists for such activities.

The number of interventions documented in this pilot project are indicative of the breadth and depth of pharmacist involvement in solving other drug related problems with geriatric patients' therapies. At present these cost savings are unrecognized and certainly not reimbursed.

The total amount of estimated intervention cost savings is a substantive amount. This amount is probably an underestimate of costs saved. Several of the pharmacists were reluctant to indicate an avoided outcome due to their interventions. Because of lack of reimbursement for such activities, pharmacists are simply not used to documenting the scope of their activities. In addition to avoidance of major dollar expenditures, the savings attributable to generic or therapeutic substitution, drug discontinuance, or non-filling of prescriptions was sizable.

The results of this project are indicative of the enormous scope of pharmacists' activities which, although currently unreimbursed, make a tremendous positive impact upon the therapeutic and economic well-being of patients. It must be noted that the pharmacists who participated in this study had not received formal training in documenting interventions. The one page directions for filling out the intervention form was a very rudimentary introduction into the procedures for filling out this particular form. With further education and training in documenting, no doubt the number and quality of the documented interventions would increase dramatically. Further efforts need to be undertaken to document pharmacist activities which profoundly benefit patients and other professionals in the health care milieu, and result in significant cost savings to the health care system.

REFERENCES

1. Bootman JL. Application of cost benefit analysis to community pharmacy practice. *Canadian Pharmacy Journal* 1986; 119: 295-296, 298, 300-303.

2. Community practice study shows pharmacist interventions add economic value to patient care. *American Journal of Hospital Pharmacy* 1991; 48: 1376, 1380.

3. Moss RL, Henderson RP, Burke JM et al. Documenting the activities of clinical pharmacists. *American Journal of Hospital Pharmacy* 1988; 45: 621-622.

4. Bussieres JF, Lepage Y. Reduction of costs and drug consumption in prolonged care through the impact of a pharmacist. *Canadian Journal of Hospital Pharmacy* 1991; 44(3): 121-129.

5. Davis KR, Allen KL. Poster Presentation. Financial impact of routine pharmacist intervention in a managed care system. ASHP Midyear Clinical Meeting 1990; 25: HMO-06.

6. USP Conference addresses the role of patient education. *American Journal of Hospital Pharmacy* 1992; 49: 2871-2873.

7. Stephens MA, Ryan MR, Gourley DR et al. Poster Presentation. Economic impact of a retrospective chart review program in an adult medicine clinic. ASHP Midyear Clinical Meeting 1992; P-448R.

8. Hatoum HT, Witte KW, Hutchinson RA. Patient care contributions of clinical pharmacists in four ambulatory care clinics. *Hospital Pharmacy* 1992; 27: 203-206, 208-209.

9. Wertheimer AI. Managed care pharmacy service. *Topics in Hospital Pharmacy Management* 1990; 10: 1-7.

10. Christensen DB, Fassett WE, Andrews GA. A practical billing and payment plan for cognitive services. *American Pharmacy* 1993; Vol. NS 31, No. 3: 34-40.

11. Fincham JE, Hospodka RJ, Scott DM. The true value of pharmacist care. *NARD Journal*, Vol. 17, No. 3, 29-31, 1995.

12. Rupp MT, DeYoung M, Schondelmeyer SW. *Prescribing Problems and Pharmacist Intervention in Community Practice: A Multicenter Study.* Washington, DC: APhA Foundation; 1991.

13. *1995 Physician Fee & Coding Guide.* Augusta, GA: HealthCare Consultants of America, Inc., 1995.

14. *American Hospital Association, American Hospital Association Hospital Statistics 1992-1993 Edition* Chicago, Illinois: American Hospital Association, 1992.

15. *The Medicare DRG Handbook, Comparative and Financial Standards,* Baltimore, Maryland: Health Care Investment Analysts, Inc., Cleveland, Ohio: Ernst & Young, 1991.

APPENDIX A. Documenting the Worth of Pharmaceutical Services: Data Collection Sheet

1. PRESCRIPTION INFORMATION

Date_____ Time of Day_____am/pm   Rx Number_____RPh Initial_____.

PRESCRIPTION STATUS	PRESCRIPTION SOURCE	PRESCRIBER TYPE
☐New R	☐Patient	☐MD
☐Refill R	☐Doctor Phoned R In	☐DO
☐Other (Specify):	☐Nurse/Secretary Phoned R In	☐DDS
_____.	☐Other (Specify):	☐DPM
	_____.	☐ARNP
		☐PA
		☐Unknown

PATIENT SEX	PATIENT AGE___yrs.	PAYMENT SOURCE
☐Female		☐Private Pay
☐Male		☐Medicaid
		☐Third Party

2. REASON FOR INTERVENTION (CHECK ALL THAT APPLY)

☐PRESCRIBING ERROR
- ☐Inappropriate Drug/Indication
- ☐Inappropriate Dose/Regimen/Strength
- ☐Inappropriate Dosage Form
- ☐Inappropriate Quantity/Duration
- ☐Incorrect Patient

☐DRUG THERAPY MONITORING
- ☐Side Effects/Toxicity/Allergic Reaction
- ☐Duplicate Therapy
- ☐Overutilization
- ☐Underutilization
- ☐Patient Concern/Question
- ☐Patient Counseling
- ☐Compliance Intervention

☐PRESCRIPTION OMISSION
- ☐Drug Not Specified
- ☐Dose/Regimen Not Specified
- ☐Form/Strength Not Specified/Unavailable
- ☐Quantity/Duration Not Specified
- ☐Incomplete Directions for Use
- ☐Illegible
- ☐Violates Legal Requirement

☐DRUG INTERACTION
- ☐R - OTC
- ☐R - R
- ☐Allergy/Sensitivity
- ☐Drug - Disease
- ☐Other (Specify)

_____.

3. DRUG(S) INVOLVED:
List Drug Name
1._____.
2._____.

4. INFORMATION SOURCES USED
(Check all that apply)
- ☐Patient Profile Consulted
- ☐Patient Interviewed
- ☐Patient Representative Interviewed
- ☐Prescriber(s) Contacted (How Many?) _____
- ☐Prescriber's Nurse/Secretary Contacted
- ☐Drug Information Source(s) Consulted
  Specify:_____.

5. PRESCRIPTION OUTCOMES
(Check all that apply)
- ☐R Dispensed as Written
- ☐R Clarified and Dispensed
- ☐R Changed and Dispensed
- ☐R Not Dispensed
- ☐Other (Specify)

_____.

APPENDIX A (continued)

6. DIRECT INTERVENTION TIME (Actual Pharmacist Contact)
With Patient or Patient Representative   _____minutes
With Other (Prescriber, Profile Review, Research) _____minutes

7. POSSIBLE THERAPEUTIC OUTCOME AVOIDED	**8. COST SAVINGS IF APPLICABLE (INDICATE AMOUNT)**
☐Emergency Room Visit	☐Generic Substitution $_____.
☐Physician Visit	☐Therapeutic Substitution $_____.
☐Hospitalization	☐Drug Discontinued $_____.
	☐Drug Not Dispensed $_____.

APPENDIX B. Documenting the Worth of Pharmaceutical Services: Data Collection Sheet Instructions

1. Please begin to fill out the data collection forms beginning the day that you receive this packet.

2. Read the intervention form completely before beginning to record interventions so that you can familiarize yourself with all the types of interventions to be recorded.

3. Fill out one form for each intervention that you make in a patient's drug therapy at the time you are actually intervening.

4. Please check the appropriate boxes on the attached sheet based upon what you have done in the intervention. You do so many things on a routine basis, but even though they seem routine to you, it is important that we document as many of these as possible.

5. If possible, please fill out **Item 6** (intervention time), **Item 7** (your assessment of a negative therapeutic outcome which was avoided by your action), and **Item 8** (the cost savings that you estimate to be saved by your actions).

6. If you can be more detailed about your intervention—that is great. Please write more detailed explanations on the back of the form if you need to, but if you would prefer to check only the categories on the front of the sheet—that is okay too.

7. An example of an intervention is attached, please use it as a guide for completing the sheets. The more complete and specific that you can be when recording this data will allow us to obtain better results.

8. At the end of each of the four weeks, please mail the completed forms back to us in the postage paid envelope. If you need more forms, please call us and we will send them to you.

9. All information that we will collect will be held in the strictest confidence.

10. Please contact Jack Fincham (913) 864-3591 if you have any questions.

Thank you for your help. It is much appreciated!

APPENDIX C. Drugs Mentioned on the Intervention Data Sheets

Gastrointestinal

Pepcid AC ™	2
Propulsid ™	1
Donnatal ™	1
Pepto Bismol ™	2
Tagamet ™	1
Prilosec ™	1
Docusate	1
Donnazyme ™	1

Anti-infectives

Amoxicillin	2
Cephalexin	3
Biaxin ™	1
Cipro ™	4
Ceclor ™	1
Diflucan ™	1
Sporanox ™	3
Doxycycline	2
Penicillin	1
Suprax ™	1
Nystatin Oral	2
Tetracycline	1
Rocephin ™	1

NSAIDs

Daypro ™	1
Naproxen	4
Relafen ™	1
Cataflam ™	1
Lodine ™	1
Indocin ™	1
Piroxicam	1

Analgesics

Lortab ™	4
Tylenol #3 ™	3
Duragesic ™	4
Darvocet N-100 ™	2
Trilisate ™	2
Ecotrin ™	1
Morphine Sulfate	1

Hyperlipidemia

Gemfibrozol	1
Questran ™	2
Colestid ™	1

Ophthalmics

Timoptic ™	2
Gentamicin	2
Maxitrol ™	1
Viroptic ™	1
Trusopt ™	1
Flarex ™	1
Betagan .5% ™	1
Blephamide ™	1

Products

Blood Glucometer	1

Benzodiazepines/Antianxiety

Xanax ™	1
Lorazepam	1
Diazepam	3
Klonopin ™	1
Ambien ™	1
Oxazepam	2
Temazepam	1
Vistaril ™	1
Tranxene ™	1
Halcion ™	1
Buspar ™	1
Dalmane ™	1

Antidepressants

Amitriptyline	3
Sinequan ™	2
Pamelor ™	1

Other Psychotropics

Dexedrine ™	1

Topicals

Lidex ™	1
Diprolene ™	2
Cortaid ™	1
Proctocream ™	1
Synalar ™	1
Cyclocort Cream ™	1
Diprosone Cream ™	1
Capsaicin	1
Zinc Oxide	1
Epsom Salts	1

APPENDIX C (continued)

Antidiabetic Agents

Insulin	3
Glucophage ™	4
Glynase ™	2
Diabeta ™	2
Glucotrol ™	2
Chlorpropamide	1

Cardiovascular

Coumadin ™	2
Lanoxin ™	3
Furosemide	3
Hytrin ™	2
Procardia XL ™	3
Verapamil	1
Vasotec ™	4
Propranolol	2
Lotensin ™	1
Atenolol ™	1
Dilacor ™	1
Zestril ™	1
Aldactazide ™	1
Norvasc ™	1
Minitran ™	1
Transderm Nitro ™	1
Nitro Dur ™	1
Quinidex ™	1
Dyrenium ™	1
Prazosin	1
Levatol ™	1
Lozol ™	1

Sex Hormones

Provera ™	3
Premarin ™	2

Adrenal Corticosteroids

Prednisone	1
Hydrocortisone	2

Nutritional Supplements

Potassium	5
Vitamin B6	1

Antiasthmatics/Respiratory Tract

Azmacort ™	1
Serevent ™	1
Vancenase AQ ™	1

Antihistamine/Cough & Cold

Seldane ™	1
Tessalon Pearls ™	2
Humibid LA ™	1

Antiemetic/Antivertigo

Tigan ™	1
Antivert ™	1
Meclizine	1

Other

Calcimar ™	1
Quinamm ™	2
Ditropan ™	1
Didronel ™	1

Pharmaceutical Care Provided by Doctor of Pharmacy Clerkship Students in Geriatric Patients in an Acute Care Setting

Marie A. Chisholm
A. Thomas Taylor
David W. Hawkins

SUMMARY. This study was undertaken to evaluate the pharmaceutical care provided for geriatric patients by Doctor of Pharmacy (Pharm.D.) students on clerkships. Objectives of the study included: (1) teaching pharmacy students to identify, document, solve, and prevent medication-related problems; (2) documenting the number

Marie A. Chisholm, PharmD, is Clinical Assistant Professor of Pharmacy Practice, The University of Georgia College of Pharmacy, Athens, GA 30602 and Assistant Adjunct Professor of Medicine, Medical College of Georgia, School of Medicine, Augusta, GA 30912. A. Thomas Taylor, PharmD, is Associate Professor of Pharmacy Practice, The University of Georgia College of Pharmacy, Athens, GA and Clinical Professor, Departments of Medicine and Family Medicine, Medical College of Georgia, School of Medicine, Augusta, GA. David W. Hawkins, PharmD, is Professor of Pharmacy Practice and Assistant Dean, The University of Georgia College of Pharmacy, Athens, GA and Clinical Professor of Medicine and Assistant Dean for Clinical Pharmacy, Medical College of Georgia, School of Medicine, Augusta, GA.

Address correspondence to: Marie A. Chisholm, PharmD, Medical College of Georgia, Clinical Pharmacy Program, CJ-1020, Augusta, GA 30912-2390.

[Haworth co-indexing entry note]: "Pharmaceutical Care Provided by Doctor of Pharmacy Clerkship Students in Geriatric Patients in an Acute Care Setting." Chisholm, Marie A., A. Thomas Taylor, and David W. Hawkins. Co-published simultaneously in *Journal of Geriatric Drug Therapy* (The Pharmaceutical Products Press, an imprint of The Haworth Press, Inc.) Vol. 11, No. 4, 1997, pp. 43-50; and: *Geriatric Drug Therapy Interventions* (ed: James W. Cooper) The Pharmaceutical Products Press, an imprint of The Haworth Press, Inc., 1997, pp. 43-50. Single or multiple copies of this article are available for a fee from The Haworth Document Delivery Service [1-800-342-9678, 9:00 a.m. - 5:00 p.m. (EST). E-mail address: getinfo@haworth.com].

43

and types of recommendations made by Pharm.D. students; (3) determining the physician-acceptance rate of these suggestions; (4) determining the potential impact of students' recommendations on patient care; and (5) comparing students' recommendations for geriatric patients to non-geriatric patients. Fifteen Pharm.D. students enrolled at the University of Georgia College of Pharmacy assigned to general medicine or family medicine teams at the Medical College of Georgia Hospital during July 1995 through March 1996 participated in the study. Of the 174 recommendations that were made, 57 recommendations concerned patients greater than 65 years of age. Fifty-one (89.5%) of these recommendations were accepted by physicians. Improper medication selection, untreated indication, and overdosage prompted more than half of these recommendations. The most frequent medication classifications for accepted recommendations were the anti-infective (25.5%), cardiovascular (23.5%), and gastrointestinal (13.7%) classes. Two pharmacists evaluated each accepted recommendation by using Hatoum's criteria for assessing potential impact on patient care and indicated that approximately sixty-five percent of the accepted recommendations were considered significant (56.9), very significant (5.9%), or extremely significant (2%). The authors conclude that pharmacy students can have a positive impact on geriatric patient care in an acute care environment. *[Article copies available for a fee from The Haworth Document Delivery Service: 1-800-342-9678. E-mail address: getinfo@haworth.com]*

KEYWORDS: pharmacists, care, students, geriatric, acute care

INTRODUCTION

In order to nurture the development of pharmaceutical care, pharmacy educators and practitioners must teach pharmacy students to provide patient-focused care and assume responsibility for patient outcomes. Clinical clerkship rotations in Doctor of Pharmacy (Pharm.D.) curricula provide students excellent opportunities to learn and implement pharmaceutical care under the direct supervision of an experienced practitioner. Furthermore, clerkship experiences should be evaluated by pharmacy educators and preceptors to determine the quality of clinical outcomes for the patients involved.

Pharmaceutical care is defined as the "responsible provision of medication therapy for the purpose of achieving definite outcomes that improve a patient's quality of life."[1] Furthermore, pharmaceutical care involves pharmacists establishing relationships with patients and other professionals in designing, implementing, and monitoring a therapeutic plan that will provide specific therapeutic outcomes.[1] Although the concept and importance of pharmaceutical care have been described in the literature, there are no published data describing pharmaceutical care provided by pharmacy students in a geriatric population. Therefore, the purpose of this study was to evaluate the pharmaceutical care activity in geriatric patients provided by Pharm.D. students assigned to acute care clinical rotations. The study published in *Hospital Pharmacy*,[2] provided the impetus for this follow-up study reporting the provision of pharmaceutical care in the acute care geriatric patient population. The objectives of the study were to: (1) teach pharmacy students to identify, document, solve, and prevent medication-related problems; (2) document the number and types of recommendations made by Pharm.D. students; (3) determine the physician-acceptance rate of these suggestions; (4) determine the potential impact of students' recommendations on patient care; and (5) compare students' recommendations for geriatric patients to non-geriatric patients.

METHODOLOGY

Of the fifteen Pharm.D. students participating in this study, eleven were enrolled in the entry-level program. Four students had previously received a baccalaureate pharmacy degree. During July 1995 through March 1996, these students were assigned to a 4-week clerkship with a general medicine or a family medicine team at the Medical College of Georgia (MCG) Hospital, a 540-bed tertiary-care teaching facility located in Augusta, Georgia. Students assigned to a general medicine clerkship spent the entire 4-week clerkship on the inpatient service; students assigned to the family medicine clerkship spent two weeks on the inpatient service and two weeks in the family medicine outpatient clinic. After receiving information concerning the provision of pharmaceutical care and a standardized method to document their activities, students were encouraged to participate in all inpatient pharmacotherapy decisions during the assigned rotation.

Students conducted an initial pharmacy evaluation of each patient within 48 hours of hospital admission. This initial assessment involved consideration of medication-induced disorders and evaluation of appropriateness of medication regimens. Each student participated in daily medical rounds and patient care discussions. Specific student responsibilities, under the direct supervision of the preceptor, included identifying, resolving, and preventing medication-related problems. Therapeutic recommendations, including dosage adjustments, were based on patient-specific pharmacodynamic and pharmacokinetic parameters. Students participated in the overall management of patients throughout their hospitalization or until the end of the clerkship experience.

Students documented all pharmacotherapy recommendations throughout the clerkship using a standardized pharmacy intervention form. Students presented their findings, assessments and recommendations to the pharmacy preceptor. Each patient's medical history, hospital course, health status, and therapeutic monitoring plan were also discussed. Following this review, students communicated recommendations to the appropriate medicine interns or residents. Students noted on the intervention form whether a recommendation was accepted or rejected. The clinical results of each accepted recommendation were also recorded.

At the end of each clerkship, all pharmacotherapy recommendations were grouped into one of eight previously defined medication-related categories (Table I).[3] Each recommendation was further categorized into specific medication classifications. Each accepted recommendation was independently ranked and scored by a preceptor and a practicing pharmacist according to its potential impact on patient care using Hatoum's criteria[4] and the point scale illustrated in Table II. Average significance scores for all accepted recommendations were calculated by adding the significance scores of all accepted recommendations and dividing by the total number of recommendations.

RESULTS

Fifteen students participated in this study, making 174 recommendations in 110 general medicine or family medicine patients. Of these recommendations, 150 (86.2%) were accepted by the medical team. Of the 174 recommendations, 57 recommendations were for patients greater than 65 years old (32 patients). Fifty-one (89.5%) of

TABLE I. Medication-Related Problem Category

Untreated Indication	The patient has a medical problem that requires medication therapy (an indicator for medication use) but is not receiving a medication for that indication.
Improper Medication Selection	The patient has a medication indication but is taking the wrong medication. This includes allergy to the medication and availability to a less expensive, equally effective medication therapy.
Subtherapeutic Dosage	The patient has a medical problem being treated with too little of the correct medication.
Failure to Receive Medication	The patient has a medical problem that is the result of his or her not receiving a medication.
Overdosage	The patient has a medical problem that is being treated with too much of the correct drug (toxicity).
Adverse Drug Reactions	A medical problem has the potential to develop or has already developed that is the result of an adverse effect.
Medication Interactions	The patient has a medical problem that is the result of a drug-drug, drug-food, or drug-laboratory interaction.
Medication Use Without Indication	The patient is taking a medication for no medically valid indication or a therapeutic medication duplication exists in which one medication should be effective.

[3]Strand LM, Morley PC, Cipolle RJ, Ramsey RR et al. Drug-related problems: their structure and function. DICP Ann Pharmacother. 1990;24:1093-71.

the 57 recommendations for the elderly patients were accepted. Improper medication selection, untreated indication, and overdosage accounted for greater than half of the medication-related problems (Table III). The most frequent medication classifications for accepted recommendations were the anti-infective (25.5%), cardiovascular (23.5%), and gastrointestinal (13.7%) classes (Table IV). Approximately, sixty-five percent of the accepted recommendations were considered significant (56.9), very significant (5.9%), or extremely significant (2%) with an average significance score of 2.22 (Table V). Tables III, IV, and V contain comparative data between the geriatric and non-geriatric patients included in the study.

TABLE II. Recommendation Significance Scale

Score	Significance	Definition
−1	Adverse Significance	Recommendation may lead to adverse outcomes
0	No significance	Recommendation is informational (not specifically related to the patient in question)
1	Somewhat significant	Benefit of the recommendation to the patient could be neutral depending on professional interpretation
2	Significant	Recommendation would bring care to a more acceptable and appropriate level
3	Very significant	Recommendation qualified by a potential or existing major organ dysfunction
4	Extremely significant	Information qualified by life and death situation

[4]Hatoum HT, Hutchinson RA, Witte KW et al. Evaluation of the contribution of clinical pharmacists: inpatient care and cost reduction. Drug Intell Clin Pharm. 1988; 22:252-9.

Table III. Medication Recommendation Category

Type of Medication-Related Recommendations	Geriatric No. (%)		Non-Geriatric No. (%)	
Improper medication selection	17	(33.3)	16	(16.2)
Overdosage	8	(15.7)	21	(21.2)
Untreated indication	7	(13.7)	22	(22.2)
Adverse Drug Reactions	7	(13.7)	14	(14.1)
Medication use without an indication	6	(11.8)	6	(6.1)
Subtherapeutic dosage	2	(3.9)	17	(17.2)
Drug-drug interaction/drug-food interaction	2	(3.9)	2	(2)
Failure to receive medication	2	(3.9)	1	(1)
Total	51	(100)*	99	(100)*

*Rounded to the nearest whole number.

TABLE IV. Medication Classification of Recommendations

Classifications	Geriatrics No. (%)	Non-Geriatrics No. (%)
Anti-infective	13 (25.5)	43 (43.4)
Cardiovascular	12 (23.5)	17 (17.2)
Gastrointestinal	7 (13.7)	9 (9.1)
Electrolyte, caloric, and H_2O balance	6 (11.8)	8 (8.1)
Analgesics	2 (3.9)	0 (0)
Miscellaneous*	11 (21.6)	22 (22.2)
Total	51 (100)	99 (100)*

*Miscellaneous classification includes hormones and synthetic substitutes, vitamins, anticonvulsants, antidiabetics, chemotherapeutic, sedatives, and psychotherapeutic agents.

TABLE V. Significance of Recommendations

Interval Score	Classification	Geriatric No. (%)	Non-Geriatric No. (%)
0.5-0.9	No significance	0 (0)	1 (1)
1.0-1.9	Somewhat significant	18 (35.3)	29 (29.3)
2.0-2.9	Significant	29 (56.9)	51 (51.5)
3.0-3.9	Very significant	3 (5.9)	17 (17.2)
4.0	Extremely significant	1 (2)	1 (1)
	Total	51 (100)*	99 (100)

*Rounded to the nearest whole number.

DISCUSSION AND CONCLUSION

The primary purpose of this study was to evaluate pharmaceutical care activity performed by clerkship students in acute care geriatric patients. Results indicate that students actively participated in patient care by identifying and resolving medication-related problems. An average of 1.78 recommendations were made for each geriatric patient and an average of 1.78 recommendations involving geriatric patients were made by each Pharm.D. student.

Of the 57 pharmacotherapy recommendations presented to physicians, 51 were accepted. The acceptance rate of 89.5% in the elderly patients was slightly higher than the 84.6% in the non-geriatric population. These acceptance rates are also slightly higher than the 85.5% reported in the literature for recommendations made by practicing pharmacists.[4]

The potential impact of the interventions in this study was determined by taking the average combined impact scores of the practicing pharmacist and the clerkship preceptor using Hatoum's scale (Table II). All of the accepted recommendations were considered to be at least somewhat significant (Table V). Approximately 8% of the recommendations were judged to have a very significant or extremely significant impact on geriatric patient care. As cited in *Hospital Pharmacy,*[2] most of the interventions classified as having a significant, very significant, or extremely significant potential impact on patient care involved changing to an appropriate antibiotic or making a dosage adjustment of a medication for organ dysfunction. The one extremely significant intervention involved a heparin overdosage. According to the average accepted recommendation significance score of 2.22, most recommendations were considered to have a significant impact on patient outcomes as judged by a practicing pharmacist and a pharmacy preceptor. Therefore, with proper supervision, pharmacy students can have a positive impact on geriatric patient care through individualized pharmacotherapeutic interventions.

REFERENCES

1. Hepler CD and Strand LM. Opportunities and responsibilities in pharmaceutical care. Am J Hosp Pharm. 1990; 47:533-43.

2. Chisholm MA, Hawkins DW, and Taylor AT. Providing pharmaceutical care: are pharmacy students beneficial to patients? Hosp Pharm. 1997;32:370-375.

3. Strand LM, Morley PC, Cipolle RJ, Ramsey RR et al. Drug-related problems: their structure and function. DICP Ann Pharmacother. 1990;24:1093-7.

4. Klopher JD, Einarson TR. Acceptance of pharmacists suggestions by prescribers: a literature review. Hosp Pharm. 1990;25:830-2, 834-6.

Consultant Pharmacist Drug Therapy Intervention Recommendations in a Geriatric Nursing Facility: A One-Year Study

James W. Cooper

SUMMARY. *Purpose*: To analyze drug therapy recommendations acceptance or rejection costs in a nursing facility practice.

Methods: Admission patient assessment, problem list and monthly problem-oriented drug regimen review (DRR) and assessment, with written report and mandated response by attending physician and follow-up on subsequent months DRR. Descriptive statistics of patient demographics and recommendation acceptance and types. Cost calculation of consequences of acceptance or rejection.

James W. Cooper, PhD, BCPS, FASCP, FASHP, is Professor of Pharmacy Practice, College of Pharmacy, and Gerontology Faculty, The University of Georgia, Athens, GA 30602, and Assistant Clinical Professor, Department of Family Medicine, Medical College of Georgia, Augusta, GA 30912.

The author is grateful to Dr. Samuel W. Kidder and Dr. Henry H. Cobb III for their review and helpful comments on this paper.

This paper was presented in part at the American College of Clinical Pharmacy Meeting, San Diego, CA, February 1994 and the Virginia chapter of the American Society of Consultant Pharmacists Meeting, Williamsburg, May 1995.

This paper was previously published as Cooper JW, "Cost-Benefit Analysis of Consultant Pharmacist Drug Therapy Recommendations from Monthly Drug Regimen Reviews in a Geriatric Nursing Facility: A One-Year Study." J. Pharmacoepidemiology 1997; 6(1): 23-36. © The Haworth Press, Inc., 1997.

Summary of Results: In 182 predominantly female patients (age 83.7 ± 7.8 years), with 4.5 ± 1.3 active problems per patient, 2004 monthly drug regimen reviews resulted in 173 recommendations in 104 (57.1%) patients. Almost 93% of the recommendations were accepted. In decreasing rank order, recommendations were for adverse drug reaction and interaction detection and resolution (47), needed nutritional or drug therapy (34), Omnibus Budget Reconciliation Act (OBRA) 1987-mandated psychotropic drug changes (32), recommended changes in dosing interval, dosage form, or administration technique (31) and lack of need, efficacy and drug duplication recommendations (29). The cost-benefit saving (ratio) from recommendation acceptance was $43,854 (4/1) or $241 per patient; the presumed cost-benefit lost by rejection was $60,825 (5.6/1) or $331 per patient.

Conclusion: Geriatric long-term care patients appear to have numerous drug-related problems (DRPs) requiring unsolicited consultations. Acceptance of consultant pharmacist recommendations may influence cost of overall care. *[Article copies available for a fee from The Haworth Document Delivery Service: 1-800-342-9678. E-mail address: getinfo@haworth.com]*

KEYWORDS: consultant pharmacists, drug regimen review, nursing homes, adverse drug reactions, costs

DRUG-RELATED PROBLEMS IN NURSING HOME PATIENTS

A two-year study has found that comprehensive drug regimen review of long-term care facility patients detects a significant drug-related problem (i.e., unwanted effect of drug therapy) every other month throughout their length of stay.[1] The consultant pharmacist has been shown to decrease overall medication costs, adverse drug reactions and interactions, medication errors, hospitalization, and mortality rates of long-term care patients.[2]

When the consultant pharmacist's services are discontinued, overall drug costs and drug-related morbidity have been shown to markedly increase and subsequently decrease when consultant services are re-initiated.[3] The reduction of drug-related problems and medication-associated costs in long-term care patients is associated with increased consultant pharmacist involvement in comprehensive pharmaceutical services. Presentation and abstract publication of a portion of this study[4] from a patient population within a nursing facility over one year documented consultant pharmacist recommendations acceptance and patient outcomes. This presentation did not consider the pharmacoeconomic consequences of the data. The purpose of this study is to present the cost changes and outcomes associated with the acceptance and rejection of those recommendations.

METHODS

Institutional Review Board Human Subjects Committee approval as "Phamacoepidemiology Project" was obtained from the University. Admission patient assessment and development of comprehensive problem lists were done. Monthly problem-oriented drug regimen reviews (DRR) and assessments were made by the consultant pharmacist with a written report on all patients of attending physicians sent on a monthly basis. Assessment of mandated response by attending physician and follow-up on recommendations was made on subsequent months DRR. Descriptive statistics of patient demographics and recommendation acceptance and types were collected by the consultant pharmacist. Calculation of costs associated with recommendation acceptance and rejection were made by the consultant pharmacist from actual costs incurred within facility records.

Operational definitions were established for: adverse drug reactions (ADRs) as any unwanted effect of drug therapy and ADR significance was made via the Naranjo Algorithm;[5] needed therapy was defined as assessment of patient condition, history and direct observation of patient signs, symptoms and lab finding present or needed to complete the assessment and formulate recommendations. The Omnibus Budget Reconciliation Act (OBRA) 1987-mandated recommendations for justification of antipsychotic and anxiolytic, consideration of barbiturate and non-barbiturate sedative and hypnotics as "unnecessary drugs" were followed.[6]

The OBRA 1987 act further defined "unnecessary drugs" as any drug used when used: (1) in excessive dose (to include duplicative drug therapy); (2) for excessive duration; (3) without adequate monitoring; (4) without adequate indications for its use or (5) in the presence of adverse consequences which indicate the dose should be reduced or discontinued or (6) any combination of the above reasons.[6]

Recommended changes in dosing interval, dosage form, or administration technique were based on assessment of current agent doses and optimal regimen. Direct survey observation of nursing time involved from such recommendations was made by the consultant pharmacist.

Costs of medications or nutritional supplements added or discontinued were calculated on an annualized basis using actual or 1993 Redbook prices. Labor costs were calculated via observation of actual time observed per task at the hourly rate and annualized. Costs of laboratory tests and hospital admissions were taken from current and billed costs.

Cost-benefit analysis was defined as the ratio of drug, lab tests and drug-administration labor and hospitalization outcomes to the cost of providing consultant pharmacist services.[7]

RESULTS

The results in Table 1 indicate a predominantly female mid-80s aged population that had a mean number of active problems per patient of 4.5 (± 1.3). Over half (57.1%) of patients required an unsolicited pharmacotherapy recommendation as a result of the admission and monthly consultant pharmacist DRR during the study period. Out of 2,004 DRRs conducted over the year there were recommendations made for 173 (8.6%) of DRRs. Over 90% (160/173) of those recommendations were accepted within a 3 month period by the attending physician.

Types of pharmacotherapy recommendations (Table 2) in decreasing rank order were: adverse drug reaction and interaction detection and resolution, need for nutritional or drug therapy, Omnibus Budget Reconciliation Act (OBRA)-mandated psychotropic drug changes, recommended changes in drug source, dosing interval, dosage form, or administration technique, and lack of drug need, efficacy and drug duplication recommendations. Figure 1 illustrates some of the unsolicited drug therapy consult recommendations and outcomes.

Tables 3 and 4 list documented drug, lab test, labor costs and

TABLE 1. Patient Demographics

Number of Patients–182

Mean (± Std. Dev.) Age–83.7 years (± 7.8 years)

Sex Distribution–Female, 156 (85.7%); Male, 26 (14.3%)

Mean Number of Active Problems per Patient–4.5 (± 1.3)

Active Problems by Disease/Condition Classification in Decreasing Rank Order–Malnutrition, Psychiatric, Cardiovascular, Musculoskeletal, Gastrointestinal, Endocrine, Dermatologic, Pulmonary, Genitourinary, and Neurologic

Number of Patients Requiring an Unsolicited Pharmacotherapy Recommendation–104 (57.1%)

TABLE 2. Drug Regimen Review (DRR) Recommendations

Number of DRRs made over One-Year Period–2,004

Number of DRRs that resulted in an unsolicited pharmacotherapy recommendation–173 (8.6%)

Number of Recommendations that Were Accepted within a 3 month period by the Attending Physician–160 (92.5%)

Types of Pharmacotherapy Recommendations in Decreasing rank Order–

Adverse drug reaction and interaction detection and resolution–47

Need for nutritional or drug therapy–34

Omnibus Budget Reconciliation Act (OBRA)-mandated psychotropic drug changes–32

Recommended changes in dosing interval, dosage form, or administration technique–31

Lack of need, efficacy and drug duplication recommendations–29

outcomes evident from pharmacotherapy recommendation acceptance and rejection.

DISCUSSION

Pharmacist-conducted drug regimen reviews (DRRs) have been mandated in the nursing home since 1974.[8] Cost-benefit analysis of 23 published studies on nursing home DRRs published as of 1987 projected a net savings of 220 million dollars per year in America.[2] A meta analysis of 15 of these studies concluded that between 20 and 144 similar studies, with at least 150 patients in each study,

FIGURE 1. Examples of Accepted Pharmacotherapy Recommendations and Outcomes

Adverse drug reaction and interaction detection and resolution

"Recommend haloperidol 2mg TID tapering to discontinuance due to possible tardive dyskinesia with Abnormal Involuntary Movement Scale (AIMS) score of 22, Reisburg Global Deterioration Scale (GDS) of 5-6, 4 falls with 2 ER visits, and increased confusion reaction"—**OUTCOME:** Two weeks after haloperidol was tapered to discontinuance, GDS assessment now 3-4. No falls noted for 3 months after discontinuance of haloperidol.

Need for nutritional or drug therapy

"Pt. is underweight with stage III pressure ulcer and has serum albumin (SA) 2.9; recommend high protein and carbohydrate supplemental feedings with B complex, C and zinc supplement BID for foot decubitus healing"—**OUTCOME:** Stage III pressure ulcer healed within 21 days and follow-up was SA = 3.5 with 7 pound weight gain two months after recommendation acceptance.

Omnibus Budget Reconciliation Act (OBRA)-mandated psychotropic drug changes

"The OBRA-1987 suggests that temazepam not be used more than 10 consecutive days, unless 3 attempts at gradual dose reduction have been unsuccessful over a 6-month period and you believe that the nightly use has improved the patient's health status. NOTE: Pt. has fallen 11 times in the past 3 months with 3 lacerations and 4 hematomas and 3 ER visits for evaluation. Please indicate your assessment of Tapering:_____/Status:_____. Thank you."—**OUTCOME:** Temazepam tapering completed with only 3 falls during the next 3 months and no fall-related injuries.

Recommended changes in drug, dosing interval, source, dosage form, or administration technique

"Pt. hospitalized for acute myocardial infarction (AMI)—returned to NH with continuous nitroglycerin (NTG) patch, 14 doses sublingual (SL) NTG noted over past week—request bedtime (HS) removal of patch order, SL NTG to bedside, and possible need for beta blocker or calcium channel blocker one hour before patch removal or continuous coverage. Please also consider acetaminophen 650mg QID in place of buffered ASA, as Hgb/Hct has dropped from 12/36 to 9/27, and $FeSO_4$ i BID for 2 months then re-check H/H."—**OUTCOME:** All recommendations accepted and no further c/o chest pain on exertion and occasional postprandial SL NTG usage for vague epigastric complaints. Hgb/Hct to 11.6/36 on 2 month recheck.

Lack of need, efficacy and drug duplication recommendations

"Amitriptyline re-started after sertraline BID which tends to increase sleep problems, especially with PM dose. Patient fell 3 times in first week after amitriptyline re-started. Amitriptyline is associated with falls and fractures. Please consider concomitant use of two antidepressants per OBRA and suspected ADR sequence. Thank you Dr."—**OUTCOME:** On discontinuance of amitriptyline and PM sertraline improved socialization, depression scale and ADL scores with no falls were noted over the next 6 months.

with no treatment effect of DRRs, would be needed to reduce these studies to unimportant levels of effect.[9] A review of medical care in nursing homes has outlined some practical and relatively inexpensive strategies to improve the quality of care.[10] Specific methods to improve medication prescribing and utilization,[11] as well as an investigation to develop specific criteria for inappropriate medication use in nursing home residents have been published.[12]

The present study offers some further evidence of the cost-benefit (Table 5) of problem-oriented drug regimen review by the consultant pharmacist. Cost-benefit methodology[7] is based on certain assumptions to include:

1. It is possible to separate one service or intervention from another. To address the first assumption, the introduction, removal and re-introduction of DRR services within this facility has previously been shown to consecutively increase then reduce drugs, doses, adverse drug reactions and ADR-related hospitalizations.[3]

2. There is a possibility of choice between the services and interventions. The second assumption is answered by the 93% response rate to recommendations, which appears to demonstrate the choice of accepting or rejecting the recommendations; it is troubling, however that despite the low rate of rejection, the detrimental economic consequences were greater (Tables 3 and 4) for rejection than the beneficial savings for acceptance of drug therapy recommendations.

3. It is possible to estimate the outcomes associated with each service or intervention. In regards to the third assumption, the outcomes were easily quantitated, although the time estimates were tedious to gather via observation and interviews with nursing and administration.

4. It is possible to value these outcomes. In the area of value of intervention the agreement between the estimated cost of each fall ($835) by a facility administrator and a recent study of fall prevention in the community (that was not published at the time of administrator interview and survey) found that the cost per subject in the intervention group was $891.[13] The cost for preventing a fall that required medical care in the prior study (i.e., hospitalization for evaluation) was $12,392.[13] The billed cost for the fall-related hospitalizations that occurred in two present study patients with recommendations rejections despite OBRA mandate were $11,340 (for hip-nailing) and $7,840 for nosocomial pneumonia that developed

TABLE 3. Cost Analysis of Recommendations (Cases) Acceptance and Outcomes

+ = added cost in drug, lab test or labor; – = decreased cost of drug, lab test or labor; NC = no change; D/C = discontinue; WNL = within normal limits

	OUTCOMES of Acceptance and Rejection			
	DRUG	LAB TEST	LABOR	OUTCOMES
Adverse Drug Reactions/Interactions (47)				
NSAIDs Gastropathy Discontinue NSAID (10)	$ – 9960	$ – 1200	NC	No complaints of joint/muscle pain
AND Start acetaminophen (10)	$ + 1200	–	NC	
ACEI Hyperkalemia (K) or increased serum creatinine (Cr)				
Decrease dose (3) or discontinue (2)	$ – 270	$ – 465	$ – 730	K & Cr WNL
Digoxin decrease dose (4) or discontinue (1)	$ – 96	NC	$ – 146	No acute CHF
Potassium Supplement Hyperkalemia (4) D/C	$ – 480	NC	$ – 584	K = 4-5mEq/l
Hypokalemia add KCl or K-sparing diuretic (4)	$ + 678	NC	$ + 245	K = 4-5mEq/l
Warfarin dose adjustment (3)	NC	NC	NC	No DVT or CVAs nor bleeding
Antihypertensive hypotension D/C drug (2)	$ – 720	NC	$ – 292	BP < 140/90
Fluoroquinolone dose adjustment (3)	$ – 90	NC	NC	No CNS effects
Antiparkinson drug CNS effects D/C drug (2)	$ – 3100	NC	$ – 292	Improved affect
Falls from benzodiazepines (2) taper to D/C	$ – 1800	NC	$ – 292	No falls
Drug-Drug Interactions				
Antacids (A) with fluoroquinolones (4) hold A	NC	NC	NC	Infection resolved
Antacids with iron salts, pt. anemic (2) D/C A	$ – 144	NC	$ – 584	Increased hemoglobin
Multiple diuretics, D/C one (1)	$ – 120	NC	$ – 146	Dehydration resolved
Theophylline (T) with erythromycin (1) cut T dose by 1/2 for 10 days	NC	NC	NC	Infection resolved without theophylline toxicity
Total Cost Changes from ADR and recommendations accepted $20,517 – 2123 = $18,394 SAVED				
Nutritional/Drug Therapy Need				
Nutritional therapy recommended (22)	$ + 8,030	NC	NC	Incr. serum albumin
Multiple vitamin/mineral supplement (22)	$ + 262	NC	NC	Weight gain, faster healing of pressure ulcers

Recommendation				Outcome
Hematinic added in Hgb/Hct (H/H) <10/30 (8)	$+523	NC	$+1168	H/H > 10/30
Clonazepam for tertiary tardive dyskinesia (1)	$+823	NC	$+292	Able to feed, wt. gain
Antidepressant for depressive sx/depression (3)	$+2280	NC	$+438	Improved socialization affect, and orientation

Total Cost Changes from recommendations accepted $13,075 in ADDED COSTS, outcomes savings not calculated.
Legend: NC = no change; H/H = hemoglobin/hematocrit

OBRA Psychotropic Changes (32)

Taper antipsychotic or benzodiazepine (25)	$-11,820	NC	$-3650	No falls, harmful behavior nor withdrawal signs/symptoms

Total Cost Savings with recommendation acceptance = $15,470

Drug Source, Dosing Interval, Administration Changes (31)

Remove nitroglycerin patch daily (16) and	NC	NC	$+180	Incr. NTG efficacy
Add calcium channel blocker (CCB) (11) one hour before removal of patch	$+4818	NC	$+1606	No anginal attacks nor acute MIs

Total costs of recommendation acceptance $6424

Change from brand name to generic antacid (1)	$-9,600	NC	NC	No change in GI complaints
Do not crush sustained-release dosage form; change to standard release product (2)	NC	NC	NC	Avoidance of adverse effects
Change from standard to sustained-release dosage forms of diltiazem (6), nifedipine (2), verapamil (1), and propranolol (1)	NC	NC	$-4,391	Fewer administration times per day with same efficacy
Change dosing interval of antianginal from TID or QID to q 8 or q 6 hours (2)	NC	NC	NC	Consistent blood levels

Lack of Need/Efficacy (29)

Discontinue drug due to lack of need or demonstrated efficacy accepted (27)	$-7614	NC	$-7884	Fewer drugs and drug passes per patients

' Total costs saved by acceptance $15498

NET SAVINGS FROM PHARMACOTHERAPY RECOMMENDATIONS ACCEPTANCE = $43,854

TABLE 4. Cost Analysis of Recommendations (Cases) Rejection and Outcomes

Recommendation	OUTCOMES of Recommendation Rejection

Adverse Drug Reactions/Interactions (4/47 rejected)

NSAIDs Gastropathy   Discontinue NSAID
                     AND Start acetaminophen

Two NSAID-related Hospitalizations = $10,886
No Change in one patient.

Decrease dose or discontinue digoxin (1)

One hospitalization with digoxin toxicity = $+6780

Rejection $17,566 IN ADDITIONAL COSTS

OBRA Psychotropic Changes (5/32) Rejected

Taper antipsychotic or benzodiazepine

Refused to taper or withdraw in 5 with 12 falls ($835@) = 10,820 and 2 Hospital-
izations for hip fracture and pneumonia subsequent to fall at costs of $19,210

Total costs associated with recommendation refusal = $30,030

Drug Source, Dosing Interval, Administration Changes (2/31 rejected)

Remove nitroglycerin patch daily add calcium channel
blocker (CCB) hour before removal of patch

NTG patch removal/CCB addition recommendation
refused in 2 cases with one acute nonfatal MI $+12,438

Total costs of recommendation rejection = $12,438

Lack of Need/Efficacy (2/29)

Discontinue drug due to lack of need or demonstrated efficacy rejected in 2 cases = drug cost = $+480 and administration costs $+292.

Total costs savings lost by rejection cost $772.

NET COSTS ASSOCIATED WITH RECOMMENDATION REJECTION = $60,825

TABLE 5. Cost-Benefit Analysis (CBA) of Services

Cost of Consultant Pharmacist Services and Travel for one year = $10,925

Total Cost Saving Calculated for Recommendation Acceptance over one year = $43,854

Cost-Savings per patient from recommendations accepted over one year = $240.96

Cost-Benefit Ratio for Recommendation Acceptance over one year = 4.0/1

Total Presumed Costs of Recommendation Rejection over one year = $60,825

Cost-savings lost by recommendation rejection per patient over one year = $331.24

Presumed Cost Benefit Unavailable due to Rejection = 5.6/1

Total Cost Benefit if all recommendations were accepted = $104,679

Total Cost-Benefit Ratio if all recommendations accepted = 9.61

after hospitalization from the nursing home (Table 4, total $19,210). NSAID gastropathy hospitalizations[2] resulting from rejection of request to discontinue NSAIDs averaged $5,443.

An earlier study within the same facility found that over 60% of adverse drug reactions within the nursing home were preventable by attention to the patients' history and relative to absolute contraindications to drug usage.[14,15] A recent study in the same facility found that NSAIDs were the most common ADR-related hospitalization among nursing home residents.[16] While explicit criteria developed for inappropriate drug usage in nursing homes state to avoid phenylbutazone and indomethacin,[12] it may be best to avoid all NSAIDs in the nursing home resident, especially since a recent controlled study found that up to 4,000 mg of acetaminophen daily is equivalent to 1200-2400 mg of ibuprofen daily in osteoarthritic knee pain.[17] The value of quality-of-life changes nor the psychological effects of the recommendations acceptance or rejection nor outcomes were assessed.

5. It is possible to estimate the cost of providing each service or intervention. The cost of providing consultant pharmacist services was easily determined via a capitation per patient-month fee and travel over the year. The depreciated cost of a lap-top computer used for patient data base and report preparation was not included in the cost of services.

6. Costs and benefits of each service or intervention can be weighed against each other. Comparison of other similar services

was possible, as patients were seen and orders reviewed monthly to every third month by their attending physician, depending on whether patient was certified for skilled or intermediate care. When the consultant services were interrupted in this facility,[3] all associated medication costs have been shown to increase. In the present study the patient who did not have her nitroglycerin (NTG) patch removed at bedtime nor a calcium channel blocking (CCB) agent added to her therapy despite repeated anginal attacks and the recommendation for both interventions for more than 3 months, suffered a non-fatal myocardial infarction hospitalization. She has subsequently been placed on bedtime removal of the patch and a sustained-release calcium channel blocker (CCB) as well as oral beta blocker with from 0 to 5 sublingual NTG tablets used per month. A recent study has documented the contribution of the consultant pharmacist to improved diabetic patients outcomes in nursing home where recommendations are not only accepted but implemented by the consultant pharmacist under protocol with the attending physician.[18]

CONCLUSION

Geriatric patients have numerous drug-related problems (DRPs) requiring unsolicited consultations to resolve these DRPs. Considerable cost-savings may be evident when these recommendations are accepted and costs generated when the recommendations are rejected. Prevention of ADRs and adherence to the OBRA-mandated changes, as well as attention to therapeutic problems with drugs may do much to lower costs and improve the quality of drug therapy in the nursing home.

REFERENCES

1. Cooper JW. Drug-related problems in geriatric long term care facility patients. The Haworth Press, Inc., Binghamton, NY 1991.

2. Kidder SW. Cost-benefit of pharmacist-conducted drug-regimen reviews. Consult Pharm 1987;2(5):394-398.

3. Cooper JW. Effect of initiation, termination and reinitiation of consultant clinical pharmacist services in a geriatric long term care facility. Med Care 1985; 23:84-86.

4. Cooper JW. Pharmacotherapy recommendations from monthly drug regimen reviews in a geriatric nursing facility: a one year study. Pharmacotherapy 1993;13(6):687(Abstract#89).

5. Naranjo C, Busto U, Sellars E et al: A method for estimating the probability of adverse drug reactions. Clin Pharmacol Ther 1981; 30:239-45.

6. Anonymous. Omnibus budget reconciliation act of 1987. Subtitle C-Nursing home reform. Social Security Act, revised, 1987.

7. Draugalis JR et al. Pharmacoeconomics, Current Concepts, Upjohn, 1989.

8. Fed Reg, 17 Jan 74 p. 228.

9. McGhan WF, Einarson TR, Sabers DL et al. A meta-analysis of the impact of pharmacist drug-regimen reviews in long-term care facilities. J Geriatr Drug Ther 1987;1(3):23-34.

10. Ouslander JG. Medical care in the nursing home. JAMA 1989; 262:2582-2590.

11. Gurwitz JH, Soumerai SB, Avorn J. Improving medication prescribing and utilization in the nursing home. J Am Geriatr Soc 1990;38:542-552.

12. Beers MH, Ouslander JG, Rollingher I et al. Explicit criteria for determining inappropriate medication use in nursing home residents. Arch Intern Med 1991;151:1825-1832.

13. Tinetti ME, Baker DI, McAvay G et al. A multifactorial intervention to reduce the risk of falling among elderly people living in the community. N Engl J Med 1994;331:821-827.

14. Cooper JW. Drug-related problems in nursing home patients: contraindications to drug usage. Nurs Homes 1987;36(3):5-7.

15. Cooper JW. Adverse drug reactions and interactions in a nursing home. Nurs Homes 1987; 36(4):7-11.

16. Cooper JW. Adverse drug reaction hospitalizations of nursing facility residents, submitted.

17. Bradley J, Brandt K, Katz B et al. Comparison of antiinflammatory and analgesic doses of ibuprofen and acetaminophen in the treatment of patients with osteoarthritis of the knee. N Engl J Med 1991;325:87-91.

18. Cooper JW. Consultant pharmacist contribution to diabetes mellitus patient outcomes in two nursing facilities. Consult Pharm 1995;10:40-45.

CASE REPORT

Geriatric Drug Therapy Intervention Failure and Associated Costs

James W. Cooper

SUMMARY. The failure to intervene or to have intervention recommendations accepted when drug therapy problems occur in the geriatric patient can have serious personal and economic consequences. A case of both lack of intervention and failure to accept recommendations is provided by a consultant pharmacist. Intervention failure resulted in excess of $50,000 in unnecessary health system costs due to three preventable hospitalizations and a 6-month nursing facility stay. *[Article copies available for a fee from The Haworth Document Delivery Service: 1-800-342-9678. E-mail address: getinfo@haworth.com]*

KEYWORDS: geriatric, drugs, interventions, costs, pharmacist

James W. Cooper, PhD, BCPS, FASCP, FASHP, is Professor of Pharmacy Practice, College of Pharmacy, and Gerontology Faculty, University of Georgia, Athens, GA 30602, and Assistant Clinical Professor, Department of Family Medicine, Medical College of Georgia, Augusta, GA 30912.

[Haworth co-indexing entry note]: "Geriatric Drug Therapy Intervention Failure and Associated Costs." Cooper, James W. Co-published simultaneously in *Journal of Geriatric Drug Therapy* (The Pharmaceutical Products Press, an imprint of The Haworth Press, Inc.) Vol. 11, No. 4, 1997, pp. 65-70; and: *Geriatric Drug Therapy Interventions* (ed: James W. Cooper) The Pharmaceutical Products Press, an imprint of The Haworth Press, Inc., 1997, pp. 65-70. Single or multiple copies of this article are available for a fee from The Haworth Document Delivery Service [1-800-342-9678, 9:00 a.m. - 5:00 p.m. (EST). E-mail address: getinfo@haworth.com].

65

CASE

A 73 year-old caucasian female with high blood pressure (HBP) and congestive heart failure (CHF) had a prescription filled for furosemide 40mg #30, with directions to take one tablet daily, via a mail-order pharmacy, with no interaction with her pharmacist. The prescription label read "take one tablet daily." Two weeks later she has digoxin 0.25mg #30 filled with the same directions of one tablet daily filled via mail order and still has no interactions or discussion with her pharmacist. Sixty days later she has captopril 12.5mg #60 with directions to take one tablet twice a day filled after a first hospitalization for acute pulmonary edema and heart failure. The patient also has an order for sustained-release potassium chloride 10mEq #120, with directions to take two tablets twice a day filled. This potassium order was dated 60 days earlier and filled with no pharmacist interaction. No refill of digoxin nor furosemide was requested at this time, and the pharmacist did not discuss either prescription with the patient. Three weeks later the patient is again hospitalized, this time with high potassium levels and discharged to a nursing home with an order to continue all medications brought from home. All medications after the second hospitalization (captopril and KCl) were taken as ordered by refill count. The consultant pharmacist obtained a medication history via questioning the patient and examination of medication containers, as well as calling the pharmacy of record to obtain refill dates.

The medications brought from home included all above medications and were filled as ordered with no provider pharmacist questioning of any prescription order. Two weeks later the consultant pharmacist made his initial assessment and drug regimen review (DRR) of the patient and requested labs for electrolytes, digoxin level and renal function; these tests revealed high serum potassium, creatinine and digoxin levels. The patient had her digoxin held for 17 of 30 days for pulse less than 60 beats per minute (BPM).

On the basis of these labs the consultant pharmacist recommended stopping the potassium supplement, decreasing the dose of both digoxin and captopril by one-half, and re-check of levels in 30 days; the attending physician declined to accept these recommendations and the patient was hospitalized for a third time with digitalis toxicity. On re-admission to the nursing home the consultant pharmacist's recommendations were implemented, and the patients' furosemide dose was recommended to be decreased to 20mg per day. This recommendation was made subsequent to 5 hypotensive episodes and one fall that was suspected to be related to either low blood pressure and/or orthostasis (sitting or standing BP less than 120-110/60-70 mm Hg and a systolic drop of 20mm Hg or diastolic drop of 10mm Hg on change of position).

Six months later the patient is discharged from the nursing facility as she believes that she does not require this level of care, and returns to her home with quarterly calls from her consultant pharmacist to determine her medication status. Total excess costs to health care system for nursing home stay, three preventable hospitalizations, labs and medications, was in excess of $50,000.

Case Discussion—The pharmacists who filled the initial and subsequent prescriptions did not fulfill the 1993 OBRA-required offer to counsel nor determine if the patient knew when or how to take the drug or the purpose of the medication.[1] The use of mail-order pharmacy services may or may not have contributed to the problem, as it is a common observation that many community pharmacists avoid the OBRA counseling mandate, by having the pharmacy clerk ask the patient to sign a release stating that they do not want counseling.

The patient, on questioning by the consultant pharmacist, was actually taking the furosemide at bedtime and had to get up three to 5 times per night to urinate, so she stopped taking the drug after 3 doses. Two weeks later a digoxin order was filled with no questions asked; her attending physician thought the patient's heart failure had worsened, stated this to the patient and assumed that she was taking her diuretic as prescribed. The potassium chloride order was filled two months after it was issued with the captopril with no questions, even though the interaction is flagged on most all drug interaction screening programs. Digoxin was overdue for a refill, but this was not questioned.

Whether or not the patient had impaired renal function before the angiotensin converting enzyme inhibitor (ACEI) was prescribed could not be determined, but the order to continue all meds brought from home was filled, even though the patient's chart clearly stated that the discharge diagnosis from the hospital to the nursing home clearly stated the reason for the admission was due to hyperkalemia.

Once all drugs were given reliably, the underlying renal impairment of the patient made the patient's digoxin dose too high and the potassium supplement unnecessary and potentially lethal.

The prescriber failed to accept the consultant pharmacist's recommendations made in compliance with the 1987 and 1990 OBRA mandates regarding "unnecessary drugs"[2] and another hospitalization occurred. On return to the nursing facility after the third hospitalization, the recommendations were implemented, and the patient still had problems of low blood pressure. After a call was made directly to the prescriber, a recommendation to decrease furosemide dose was made by the pharmacist and accepted by the physician. When normal sinus rhythm and no atrial fibrillation were noted and the patient still had low blood pressures on 12.5mg captopril per day, the physician discontinued both digoxin and captopril.

The patient realized she did not need to be in a nursing facility and returned to her former residence on furosemide 20mg per day and is still managing her household with quarterly checkups by her physician and consultant pharmacist. This case illustrates the simple failure to ensure that the patient knew how to take the first drug for her heart failure and high blood pressure. Subsequent drugs were needlessly added and hospitalizations occurred that could have been avoided by both communications between pharmacists as the patient moved between levels of care and better physician assessment and acceptance of the pharmacist's recommendations.

Continual Pharmacy Care (CPC) is a concept proposed 22 years ago.[3] The use of CPC involves:

1. A "Continuum of Care" from patient initial assessment to;
2. Involvement in the therapy decision-making process and outcomes to;
3. Selection of modality (ies), drug, dosage form, formulation, route and system of delivery, preparation of medication for use and provision to patient/caregiver to;
4. Counseling patient or caregiver and prescriber(s) on recommended actions; and
5. Monitoring and Management of patient outcomes progress, prognosis, and drug-related problems (DRPs).

REGULATORY MANDATES FOR CONTINUAL
PHARMACY CARE

The Omnibus budget reconciliation acts of 1987 and 1990 mandate certain cognitive clinical services in the care of patients.[2] Clinical activities of the pharmacist can be viewed as a continuum of effort from the time the patient enters one's practice, whether in the community pharmacy, nursing home (facility), home health agency, hospital through periodic evaluations and subsequent "continuous" pharmacy care.

Drug-related Problems (DRPs) are two main types: misuse of medications and adverse drug reactions and interactions.[4] Drug-related Problems (DRPs) in decreasing order of incidence include: non-compliance (nonadherence) with prescribed or recommended therapy; adverse drug reaction or interactions between medications, drugs and food or drugs and laboratory tests; unnecessary or duplicative drug therapy or monitoring; and pharmacotherapy-treatable problems that are not being monitored or treated.[4]

Up to one-third of hospital[4] and one-half of nursing facility admissions[5] are associated with DRPs. Once in long-term care, two-thirds of patients have a DRP up to every other month of their stay.[6]

The key to anticipation and prevention of DRPs is the pharmacist assuming increased responsibility for therapeutic outcomes at all levels of care. The reduction of drug-related problems and medication-associated costs in patients is associated with increased pharmacist involvement in pharmaceutical care services.[7]

The methods for DRP resolution are: the patient history, intensive drug regimen review and therapeutic plan recommendations to health care clients and other providers.[7] What occurs when cognitive clinical services of drug regimen review and therapeutic consultation are removed in long-term care? Increases in drugs and doses per patient, drug-related hospital admissions and death rate are observed.[8]

The Indian Health Service (IHS) has proposed a simple method for assessment of patient knowledge of medications that could have prevented much of the unnecessary treatment seen in this case. On both initial filling and refill of medications, three simple questions are asked of the patient: can you tell me the name of your medication and what condition it is for; how are you supposed to take your medication and how is your medication treating you? In a study of DRP-related admissions to hospitals one-half of patients who had DRPs could not answer these three questions.[4] One has to wonder what adverse drug effects and associated costs might have been avoided if these simple questions had been answered when the first drug to treat this patient's problems was ordered.

REFERENCES

1. 1993 Amendment to the Social Security Act, Title XVIII and XIX, U.S. Congress.

2. Omnibus Budget Reconciliation Act of 1987 and Combined revision of 1990, U.S. Congress, Public Law 100-203.

3. Cooper JW, Frisk PA, Walchle RC. Continuous clinical pharmacy care–a method to reduce drug-related problems in the small community. J Clin Pharmacol 1975; 15:55.

4. Frisk PA, Cooper JW, Campbell NA. Community-hospital pharmacist detection of drug-related problems upon admission to small community hospitals. Am J Hosp Pharm 1977;34:738-742.

5. Cooper JW. Nursing home admission orders and the consultant pharmacist. Cons Pharm.1987; 2:152-156.

6. Cooper JW. Drug-related problems in geriatric nursing home patients, The Pharmaceutical Products Press, Binghamton NY, 1991.

7. Cooper JW. Community and Nursing Home OBRA Drug Monitoring and Patient Education Guidelines-1993, Consultant Press, 1200 Colliers Creek Rd, Watkinsville, GA 30677, 1993.

8. Cooper JW. Consultant pharmacist initiation, termination and re-initiation of services in a geriatric long-term care facility. Med Care 1985; 23:84-86.

Index

Acute care settings, 6,43-50
Adverse reactions, in nursing home
    patients, 53-62. *See also*
    Drug-related problems
Ambulatory settings
    documentation of pharmacists'
    interventions, 27-38
    drug-related problems in, 12
Angiotensin converting enzyme
    inhibitor, 67

Calcium channel blockers, 62
California, 23
Captopril case study, 66-70
Caregivers in drug misuse, 17
Chronic care, 6
Clinical outcomes. *See* Outcomes
Combined Omnibus Budget
    Reconciliation Act of 1987
    (COBRA), 17
Compliance, defined, 12
Congestive heart failure case study,
    65-70
Consultants
    cost analysis of services, 51-62
    intervention failure costs, 65-70
Continual Pharmacy Care, 68-70
Costs of health care
    adverse drug reactions, 10-11
    crisis-dominated vs. wellness
    awareness, 15-16
    for elderly, 4-5
    legislation, 17
    pharmacist interventions in
    ambulatory patients,
    29,34-35,36,37

nursing homes, 55-62
rationing care, 18-19
reimbursement for pharmacists,
    22
savings through pharmacist in
    primary care, 23
Counseling, 67

Day care patients, 11
Digoxin case study, 65-70
Disease management, pharmacist
    role in, 19-24
Doctors of pharmacy students, in
    acute care settings, 43-50
Documentation of pharmacists'
    interventions, 27-42
    benefits to patients, 28-29
    data collection sheet, 39-40
    drug related costs saved, 35,37
    drugs included, 41-42
    methods and results, 29-34
    monitoring therapy, 36-37
    reasons for, 36-38
    therapeutic outcome avoided,
    34-35,36,37
DRPs. *See* Drug-related problems
Drug abuse, 14
Drug development, 18
Drug regimen reviews, 53-57
Drug-related problems
    in ambulatory patients, 12
    defined, 5-6
    in home health and day care
    patients, 11
    in hospitals, 7
    in nursing homes, 7-11,52-62
    pharmacist interventions,
    29,34-37,46-50,52-62,69

T - #0236 - 101024 - C0 - 216/138/5 [7] - CB - 9780789003942 - Gloss Lamination